PAEDIATRIC EMERGENCIES

PAEDIATRIC EMERGENCIES

A Practical Guide to
Acute Paediatrics

Tom Lissauer, MB, MRCP

Research Fellow, Perinatal Research Unit
and Honorary Paediatric Senior Registrar,
St Mary's Hospital Medical School,
London, W2

Published, in association with
UPDATE PUBLICATIONS LTD., by

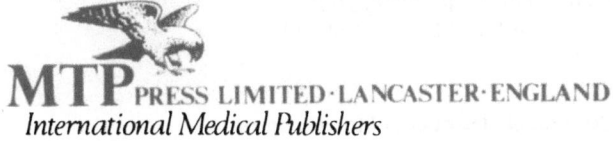

MTP PRESS LIMITED·LANCASTER·ENGLAND
International Medical Publishers

Published, in association with
Update Publications Ltd., by
MTP Press Limited
Falcon House
Lancaster, England

British Library Cataloguing in Publication Data

Lissauer, Tom
  Paediatric emergencies.
  1. Pediatric emergencies
  I. Title
  618.92′0025   RJ370

ISBN-13:978-94-009-7330-5   e-ISBN-13:978-94-009-7328-2
DOI: 10.1007/978-94-009-7328-2

Printed by **McCorquodale (Scotland) Ltd., Glasgow**

Contents

Tom Lissauer qualified from Cambridge University and University College Hospital, London, in 1973. After working as a senior house officer at The Hospital for Sick Children, Great Ormond Street, London and the Neonatal Unit at University College Hospital he spent a year in Boston at the Children's Hospital Medical Center as a Senior Resident. Since then, he has worked as Paediatric Senior Registrar at Northwick Park Hospital and Clinical Research Centre, Harrow, and at St Mary's Hospital, London. He is currently doing research in neonatal paediatrics at St Mary's Hospital Medical School, London. He is married to another paediatrician and has two young children.

Preface

The aim of this book is to provide a practical guide to help junior doctors to manage the important acute paediatric problems they are likely to encounter. The emphasis has been placed on the diagnostic problems and management when the child first presents. The approach taken is largely pragmatic, in contrast with the more theoretical approach of undergraduate teaching. As many doctors in general paediatrics are also required to perform neonatal resuscitation, a chapter on this topic has been included, but no attempt has been made to cover the specialized field of neonatal intensive care.

Several of the chapters have been published in a series of articles in *Hospital Update*. They have been thoroughly revised and many new chapters added.

It would have been impossible for me to have written this book without the help and encouragement of my wife, Dr Ann Goldman. She has read the book at each stage of its gestation and made many constructive suggestions and improvements. I am also grateful to Dr Paul Hutchins who has helped me considerably. Dr Doug Jones has provided helpful advice on the anaesthetic aspects and practical procedures and contributed the section on the insertion of central venous catheters. Many other colleagues have read sections of the book and I should like to thank Drs Ruby Schwartz, Terry Stacey, Andy Whitelaw, Rodney Rivers, John Warner, Sue Rigden, Susannah Hart, Mike Liberman and Bernard Valman. The staff of the

Update Group especially the Managing Editor Mrs Anne Patterson, the Staff Editor Sharon Kingman and Illustrator Peter Gardiner have shown me much kindness and patience. Mr Phil Johnstone of MTP Press has edited the book most efficiently. I am most grateful to Mrs Ruth White who has typed the manuscript so willingly and competently.

Photographs

I would like to thank those who have so generously allowed me to use their photographs. Their names are listed below.
Chapter 3 Figure 4: Dr R. Snook; Chapter 4 Figure 2: Health Education Council; Chapter 4 Figure 3: Department of Diagnostic Virology, St Mary's Hospital, London, W2; Chapter 5 Figure 1: Dr H. A. Davies; Chapter 8 Figure 1: Dr A. Whitelaw; Chapter 8 Figure 3: Dr Hillas-Smith; Chapter 8 Figure 4: Dr K. Rogers; Chapter 8 Figures 8, 9: Dr M. M. Liberman; Chapter 10 Figures 2, 3: Dr Vic Larcher; Chapter 14 Figures 5, 6: Radiology Department, The Children's Hospital Medical Center, Boston; Chapter 15 Figures 1, 5, 6: Dr Peter Jaffe; Chapter 15 Figures 3, 4: Dr Paul Hutchins; Chapter 15 Figure 7: Professor T. E. Oppe; Chapter 16: *Family Group* appears courtesy of the Tate Gallery, London; Chapter 17 Figures 9a and b: Dr Paul Hutchins. Kari Hutchins kindly helped drawing Figure 2 in Chapter 3.

CHAPTER 1

Neonatal resuscitation

The perinatal mortality varies considerably between westernized countries (Figure 1). Although there has been a steady reduction, lives are still undoubtedly lost and brain damage sustained because babies are still being delivered in hospitals where competent neonatal resuscitation is not always available.

Ideally, all medical members of the paediatric and obstetric staff, anaesthetists, midwives and nurses working in neonatal units should be trained and skilled in the techniques of neonatal resuscitation. Frequent changes in staff necessitate repeated lectures and demonstrations, as well as the attendance of experienced staff at deliveries until new members are confident to conduct resuscitation.

Apnoea

The sequence of events following acute total asphyxia has been extensively studied in rhesus monkeys (Dawes, 1968). There is an initial period when the animal takes rapid shallow gasps. This lasts less than a minute and is followed by a period of apnoea known as primary apnoea. After one or two minutes the animal starts to gasp again. These gasps increase in depth and frequency but then become shallow and less frequent until the last gasp. Thereafter there is no further spontaneous respiratory effort. This period of secondary or terminal apnoea ends in circulatory failure and death. In the rhesus monkey, the sequence of events up to the last gasp takes about eight minutes (Figure 2).

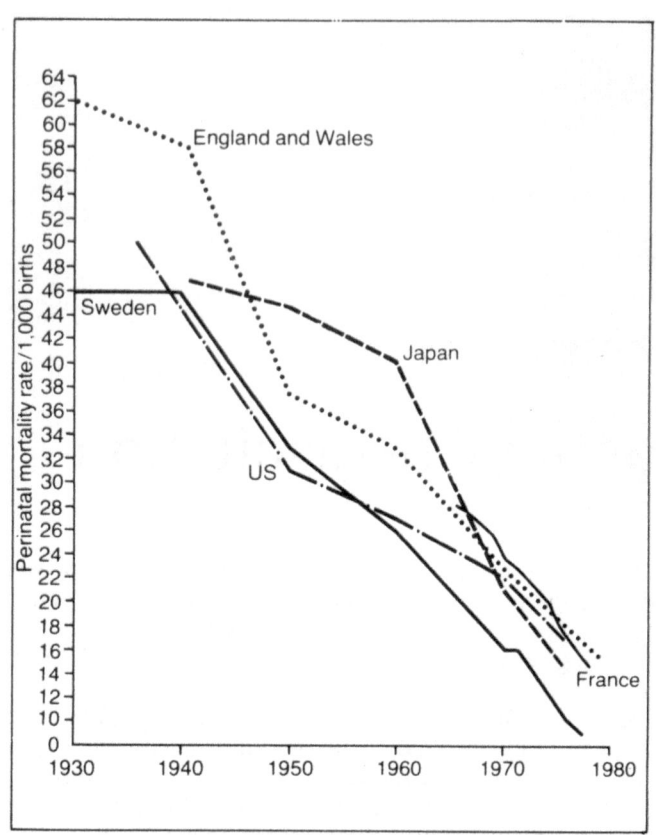

Figure 1 *Perinatal mortality in various countries*

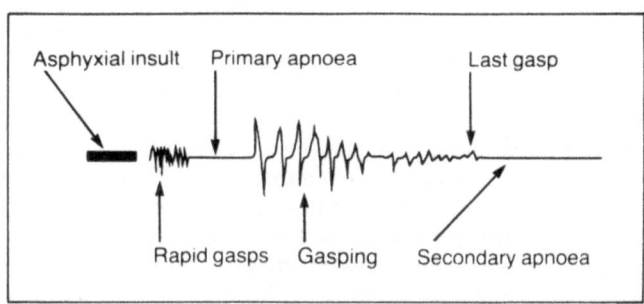

Figure 2 *Sequence of respiratory events following total asphyxia at birth in a rhesus monkey*

Primary apnoea

The human baby usually experiences intermittent partial hypoxia during labour rather than acute total asphyxia. However, the sequence of respiratory events seen in animal experiments is relevant in part to the resuscitation of the asphyxiated neonate. If there has been only minimal or moderate asphyxia the neonate may be born in primary apnoea. These babies look blue, have a heart rate greater than 100 beats per minute, and although their muscular tone is reduced there is flexion of their limbs and they make reflex responses to aspiration of their nostrils. If given appropriate stimulation regular respirations will soon follow.

Secondary apnoea

If there has been more severe asphyxia the neonate may be born in secondary apnoea. These babies look white, have a heart rate less than 100 beats per minute, and are flaccid. They do not make any reflex response to suction, and will only be successfully resuscitated if positive pressure ventilation is given. The contrasting clinical features of primary and secondary apnoea are listed in Table 1.

Table 1   Contrasting clinical features of primary and secondary apnoea

	Primary apnoea	Secondary apnoea
Heart rate	>100	<100
Colour of trunk	Blue	White
Reflex response to stimulation	Gasps or coughs	None
Posture	Flexion of limbs	Flaccid
Blood pressure	Normal or raised	Hypotension

In baby monkeys, the longer the delay in initiating resuscitation after the last gasp, the longer the time until the first spontaneous gasp. For every minute's delay in resuscitation after the last gasp, the next gasp is delayed by two minutes. The dramatic fall in heart rate following prolonged total asphyxia is shown in Figure 3. The baby monkey rapidly becomes severely acidotic from combined respiratory and metabolic acidosis. The immediate rapid elevation of P_{CO_2} from hypoventilation causes a respiratory acidosis, and the change from aerobic to anaerobic glycolysis causes a metabolic

3

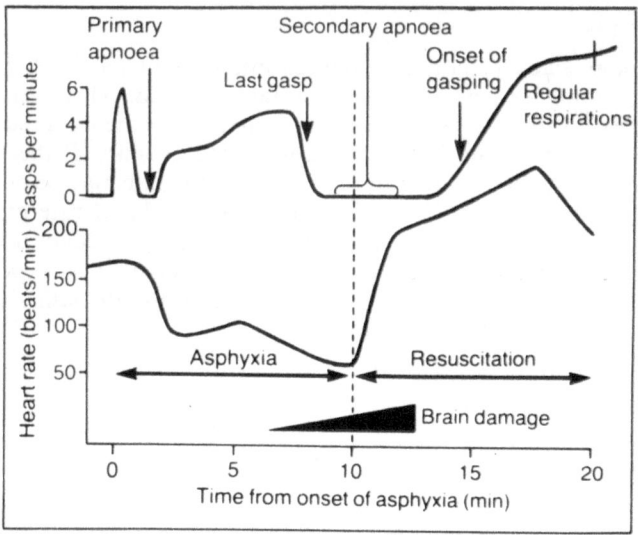

Figure 3 *Response to resuscitation in a rhesus monkey*

acidosis. After 10 minutes of total asphyxia, the pH drops from 7.3 to 6.8, the P_{CO_2} increases from 6 kPa (45 mmHg) to 20 kPa (150 mmHg) and the P_{O_2} falls from 3.4 kPa (25 mmHg) to virtually zero. Brain damage begins after approximately eight minutes of total asphyxia and is maximal after 12 to 13 minutes.

These findings emphasize the importance of rapid resuscitation of all severely asphyxiated infants. The rapid increase in the heart rate following resuscitation during secondary apnoea is also shown in Figure 3. If the heart rate is not accelerating within 30 seconds of adequate ventilation, this suggests that severe hypoxia has been sustained.

Anticipating and preparing for resuscitation

During fetal life, the lungs are filled with fluid and the circulation modified so that arterial blood from the placenta supplies the fetus with oxygenated blood. Following the transition to normal breathing at birth, the circulation has to adapt to extrauterine life, and this is triggered by tactile and thermal stimuli, as well as central chemosen-

4

sory mechanisms. Some of the reasons why a baby may fail to establish normal respiration soon after birth are listed in Table 2.

Table 2   Some causes of failure to establish normal breathing at birth

Central
Respiratory depression:
  Prolonged fetal asphyxia in labour
  Sedatives/analgesic drugs given to mother
Trauma to brain stem:
  Haemorrhage
  Herniation

Peripheral
Congenital malformations of respiratory tract:
  Pulmonary hypoplasia (often with renal agenesis, characteristic facies with prominent epicanthic folds, flattened nose and low-set ears and maternal oligohydramnios—Potter's syndrome)
  Diaphragmatic hernia
Airway obstruction

All high risk deliveries should, where possible, take place in hospitals experienced in the care of sick neonates. Regular checks should be made on fetal well-being during pregnancy and continuous fetal heart monitoring and fetal blood sampling may be employed to detect fetal distress early during labour. In many instances the need for neonatal resuscitation can be anticipated and the paediatrician called in advance (Table 3), but these criteria fail to predict the need for resuscitation in some cases, and it is imperative that a trained doctor is immediately available at all times.

Before the delivery of a baby likely to require resuscitation, the paediatrician should check that all the equipment is available and working (Figures 4 and 5 and Table 4). Details of the obstetric history, labour and, in particular, any drugs recently given to the mother should be obtained while waiting for the delivery. This can also provide an opportunity to introduce oneself to the mother and explain that one is there to look after the baby. It is always necessary to have some assistance, and for particularly high-risk infants and multiple births, the presence of an additional paediatrician is valuable.

5

Table 3   High risk deliveries

Caesarian section
Breech
Forceps delivery (except low forceps)
Multiple births
Large doses of analgesic/sedative drugs given late in labour
Fetal distress
Thick meconium in liquor
Abruptio placentae, placenta praevia
Preterm
Intrauterine growth retardation
Rhesus isoimmunization
Diabetes
Severe toxaemia
Rupture of membranes > 24 hours

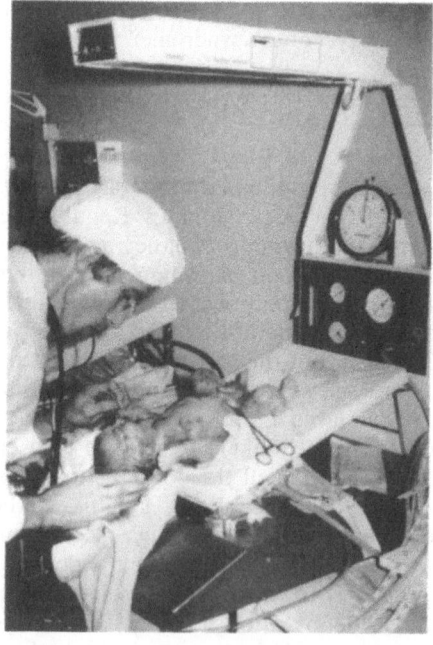

Figure 4   A resuscitaire incorporating an overhead heater and oxygen supply with pressure-gauge and suction. This new born baby's nose and mouth are being aspirated, prior to him being dried, wrapped in a warm towel and handed to his mother to hold

6

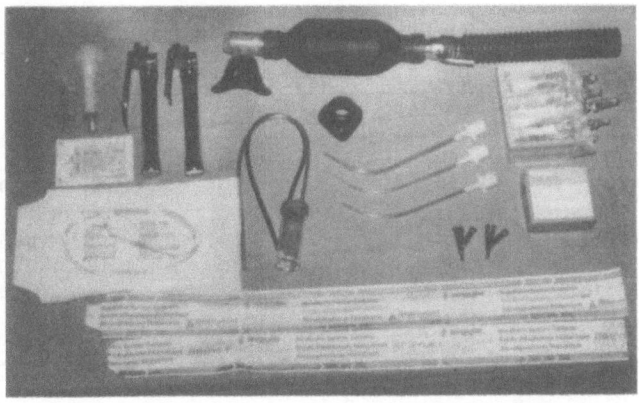

Figure 5 *Additional equipment required for neonatal resuscitation*

Table 4   Check list before delivery

1. Radiant warmer on
2. Oxygen supply and connections
3. Self-inflating bag and mask
4. Oral mucus extractor and fine suction catheters
5. Laryngoscopes with straight blades for term and preterm infants; check the light bulbs
6. Endotracheal tubes and introducer
7. Drugs: naloxone, adrenaline, dextrose, calcium chloride, sodium bicarbonate
8. Umbilical artery catheters

Apgar score

The condition of the neonate is commonly assessed using the Apgar score shown in Table 5 (Apgar, 1953). Heart rate and respiratory effort are by far the most important of the five clinical features measured, and it is these which determine the subsequent course of action. Apgar scores are routinely determined at one and five minutes. The one minute score is usually the minimum score, while the five minute score gives an impression of the infant's progress. A breakdown of how the score was derived as well as the total should always be recorded.

7

Table 5   Apgar score (modified)

	Score		
	0	*1*	*2*
Heart rate	Absent	< 100	> 100
Respiratory effort	Absent	Gasping or irregular	Regular or crying vigorously
Muscle tone	Completely flaccid	Some flexion of extremities	Well flexed with active movements
Response to nasal suction	None	Grimace	Cough or gasp
Colour of trunk	White	Blue	Pink

High risk deliveries

All newborn babies have fluid in their mouth and pharynx, which is a mixture of amniotic fluid, lung liquid and blood. Immediately after the head has been delivered the pharynx should be gently aspirated with a mucus extractor or soft suction catheter. Care should be taken not to touch the back of the pharynx as this may produce reflex bradycardia or apnoea from vagal stimulation. The clock above the resuscitaire should be started when the baby has been delivered. The infant should be placed on the resuscitaire and any remaining fluid in the mouth and nostrils gently and quickly aspirated. He should then be rapidly dried and assessed. On average, infants make their first respiratory effort within six seconds of birth, and most within 20 seconds. Rhythmic respirations have usually started by 30 seconds, but if no respiratory effort has been made by that time, active resuscitation should be started. The heart rate can be monitored either with a stethoscope on the left anterior chest wall or by palpation of the pulsation of the umbilical cord.

Most newborn babies will not need any resuscitation (Apgar score 8 to 10) and after they have been dried can be returned to their mothers.

Resuscitation

The appropriate resuscitation procedure will mainly be determined by the respiratory pattern and heart rate (Figure 6). Alternatively,

8

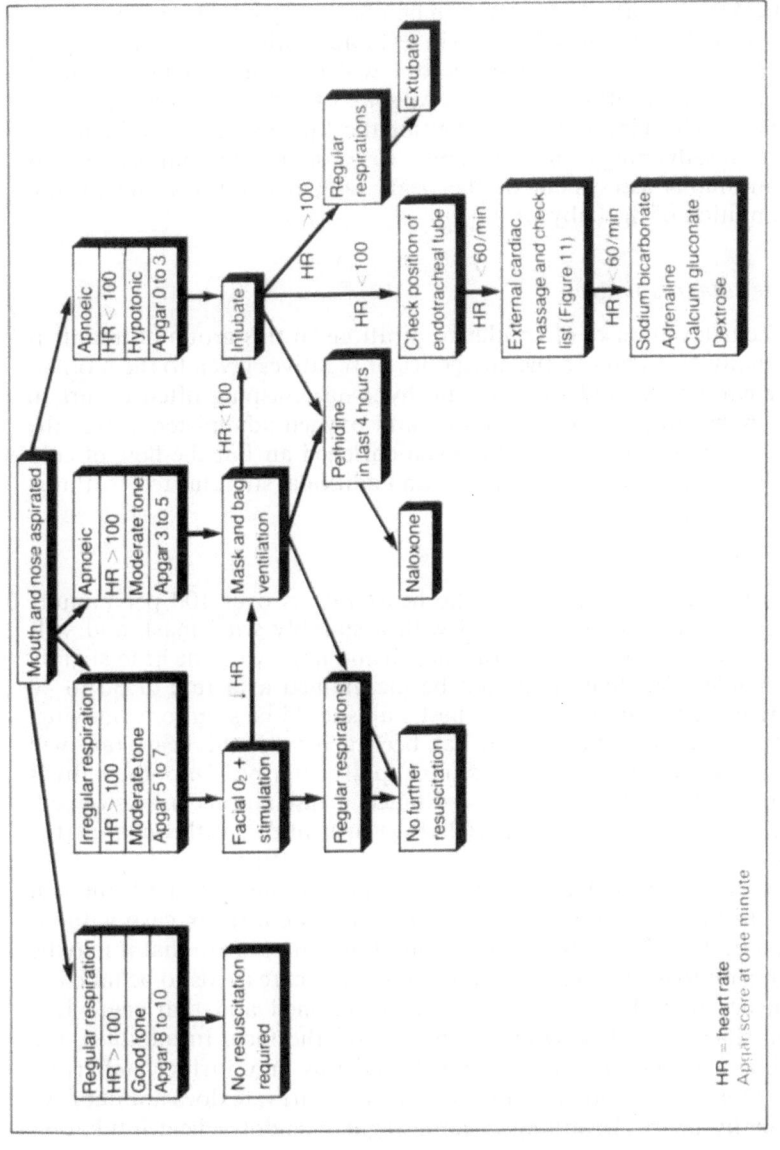

Figure 6 *Sequence for resuscitation*

9

the Apgar score at 1 minute can be used as a guide. In general those with an Apgar score of 5 to 7 will respond to stimulation and oxygen, those with an Apgar score 3 to 4 will respond to bag and mask ventilation, while those with an Apgar score of 0 to 2 need immediate endotracheal intubation. Measuring the Apgar score at 1 minute has the disadvantage that it tends to obscure the importance of continuous assessment of the heart rate, respirations and overall condition of the baby.

Irregular respiration

The delayed onset of regular respirations in this group of infants is usually secondary to the analgesics or sedatives given to the mother, or caused by mild to moderate hypoxia. Gasping often occurs in response to pharyngeal suction, and oxygen administered over the face will not only provide oxygen-enriched air but the flow of cold gas over the face will also act as an additional stimulus to breathing.

Apnoea

If the baby is apnoeic but the heart rate is over 100 per minute, ventilation should be started with a suitably sized mask and self-inflating bag applied over the mouth and nose, with the head slightly extended. Ventilation should be maintained at a rate of 30 to 40 breaths per minute and the chest wall should be seen to be moving. If satisfactory oxygenation has been achieved, the heart rate will usually accelerate and the colour rapidly improve. Once the baby is breathing regularly without assistance, resuscitation can be stopped. It is important to keep the baby warm and dry throughout the procedure.

Ventilation by bag and mask is relatively simple to perform, can be instituted rapidly and will usually initiate a reflex gasp without the trauma of intubation. Its main disadvantages are that it may be difficult to achieve effective ventilation and care needs to be taken to ensure that the head is correctly positioned and that there is a satisfactory seal between the mask and the face. In addition, the abdomen may become distended, and this may further embarrass establishing adequate respiration. If the heart rate does not improve rapidly or the breathing become regular, endotracheal intubation should be carried out.

Neonates who are apnoeic and have a heart rate less than 100 per minute should be intubated immediately. Some of them will have the clinical features of secondary apnoea (Apgar score 0 to 2). Although the Apgar score at 1 minute has been quoted, it is usually rapidly apparent that intubation is required and this should not be delayed until a minute has passed. Other babies who need intubating are those who fail to respond to bag and mask ventilation or any baby with a heart rate less than 100 beats per minute and decreasing. Babies of very low birth weight frequently require intubation. When thick meconium is present at delivery, the baby should be intubated.

Technique of intubation

The laryngoscope is held in the left hand and the blade passed over the back of the tongue bringing the epiglottis into view. It can then be advanced so that the tip lies just in front of the epiglottis (in the vallecula) and if the whole laryngoscope is lifted upwards the epiglottis swings anteriorly and the vocal cords will be visible.

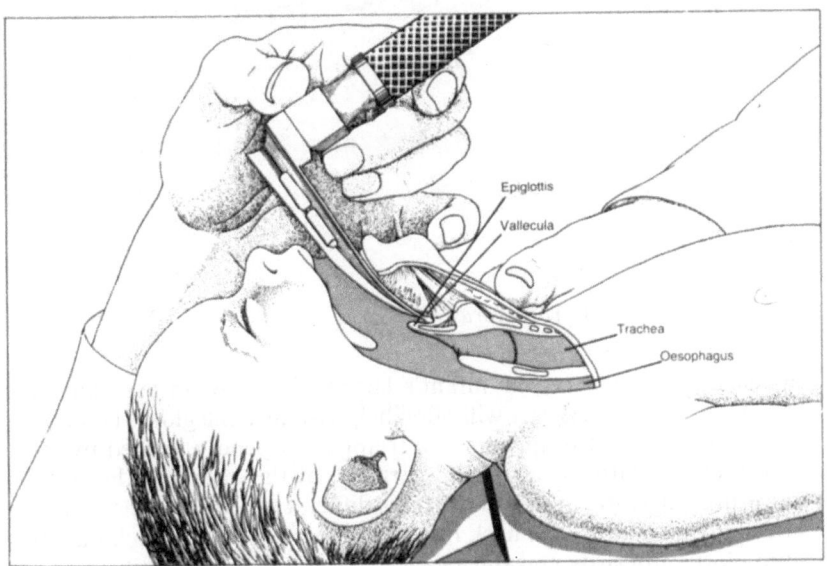

Figure 7   *Intubation of a neonate, showing the position of the laryngoscope blade*

11

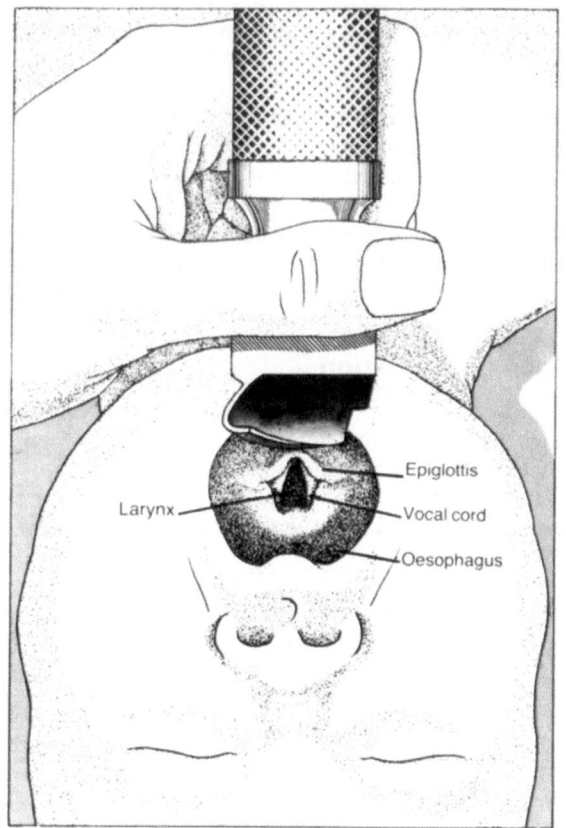

Figure 8   *View of the vocal cords*

Gentle pressure on the infant's larynx either by an assistant or with one's left little finger will often help visualize the glottis (Figures 7 and 8). The glottis appears as a triangular opening formed by the vocal cords, with the arytenoid cartilage at the base and the cords meeting anteriorly at the apex. If it is difficult to visualize the glottis, this may be because the neck has been hyperextended, which pushes the glottis upwards and out of view. This can be overcome by re-positioning the head so that it is only very slightly extended. Another problem may be that the laryngoscope blade has been inserted too

12

far, into the oesophagus, and needs to be withdrawn. In order to visualize the vocal cords it is rarely necessary to lift up the epiglottis, though this is advocated by some paediatricians. Any secretions can be quickly aspirated with a suction catheter and an endotracheal tube inserted with the right hand. The largest tube which will easily pass through the vocal cords should be used. This will vary with the size of the baby (Table 6). A soft pliable introducer may make

Table 6   Sizes of endotracheal tube

	Internal diameter
Term	3.0 mm (14 FG)
Preterm > 1000 g	2.5 mm (12 FG)
< 1000 g	2.5 mm or 2.0 mm (12 FG or 10 FG)

insertion of the endotracheal tube easier, but care needs to be taken that it does not protrude beyond the tip of the tube or it may cause damage. The endotracheal tube is inserted about 2.5 cm beyond the vocal cords in a term infant and connected via a pressure gauge to the oxygen supply (Figure 9).

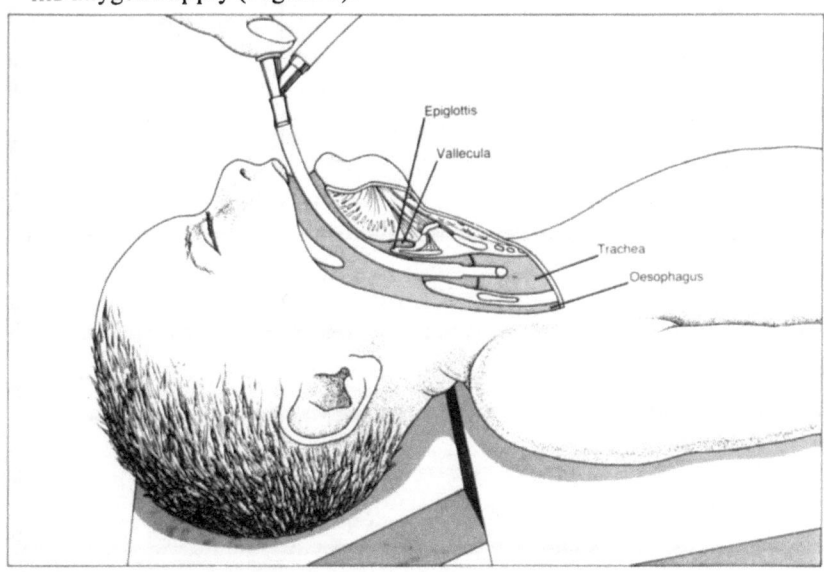

Figure 9   Endotracheal tube in position

13

Intermittent positive pressure ventilation should be started at a rate of 30 breaths per minute. The first two breaths should be at an opening pressure of $30\,cmH_2O$ (2.94 kPa) at a flow rate of 3 l/min for a term baby and held for 1 second. Subsequent breaths are at pressures of 15 to $20\,cmH_2O$ (1.47–1.96 kPa), depending on movement of the chest wall. High opening pressures for the first two breaths are needed to expand the lungs effectively, and thereafter lower pressures should be used to avoid causing a pneumothorax or pneumomediastinum. Both the intermittent positive pressure ventilation and self-inflating bag and mask should be constructed with a pressure gauge or blow-off valve so that pressures greater than $30\,cm\,H_2O$ (2.94 kPa) cannot be produced.

Difficulties with intubation

The best sign of successful resuscitation is a rapid rise in the heart rate. This is followed shortly afterwards by an improvement in col-

Problem	Signs	Action
1) Inadequate ventilation		
Faulty equipment	No air entry	Check O supply and tubing
Position of endotracheal tube:		
a) In the oesophagus	↓ Air entry ↓ Chest movement	Replace endotracheal tube
b) Down right main bronchus	Unequal breath sounds, R · L	Withdraw until breath sounds are equal
Pneumothorax	Displaced apex beat; ↓ or unequal air entry; positive transillumination	Insert butterfly needle with the other end under water or pneumothorax drain
Inadequate opening pressure	Endotracheal tube in correct position; poor chest movement	↑ Opening pressure
2) Maternal analgesia or sedation		
Has mother had pethidine or sedative drugs?	Poor respiratory effort; rapid ↑ in heart rate with ventilation	Naloxone; respiratory support
3) Shock (rare)		
Blood loss	Marked pallor when well oxygenated	Blood transfusion or plasma expander
4) Fetal abnormalities (rare)		
Hypoplastic lungs	Features of Potter's syndrome	Death inevitable
Diaphragmatic hernia	May be ventilator-dependent; scaphoid abdomen; apex often displaced	Chest radiograph; continue respiratory support; nasogastric tube

Figure 10   Check list if resuscitation is not succeeding

our, then spontaneous gasping followed by normal respiration and a gradual improvement in muscle tone. If this response is not achieved, either the infant has sustained severe intrapartum hypoxia or any of the problems listed in Figure 10 may be present. The commonest problem in achieving a successful response is incorrect positioning of the endotracheal tube and this should be checked first.

The presence of the tube in the trachea can be established by listening to the air entry over the right lateral chest wall and also by watching the chest movements. Particularly in preterm infants, sounds can be widely transmitted even if the tube is in the oesophagus, but the breath sounds will then be loudest over the stomach and there will be poor chest movements. The endotracheal tube can also easily be pushed into the right main bronchus and as this will not only reduce the oxygenation but also increase the risk of inducing a pneumothorax it is important to check that the breath sounds are equal on both sides. If there is any doubt about the position of the endotracheal tube it is often quickest to replace it. In cases of difficulty with intubation it is best not to keep trying but to stop and ventilate with a bag and mask.

External cardiac massage

External cardiac massage should be begun if the heart rate is less than 60 per minute, by using two fingers over the midsternum (Figure 11). Alternatively, an assistant can place both thumbs over the midsternum with his fingers curved around the chest, taking care to avoid pressing on the liver and abdomen (see Chapter 2, Figure 4). A suitable rate is 100 compressions per minute.

Drugs

Drugs are rarely required, as the key to successful resuscitation is ventilation of the lungs. If the infant continues to be bradycardic despite good ventilation and external cardiac massage for several minutes, sodium bicarbonate should be given. Profound metabolic acidaemia is damaging not only to the central nervous system, but also to myocardial function and causing pulmonary vasoconstriction. However, because of the dangers inherent in giving a hyperosmolar solution with a large sodium load, this should be administered only after careful consideration. It has been suggested that there is

15

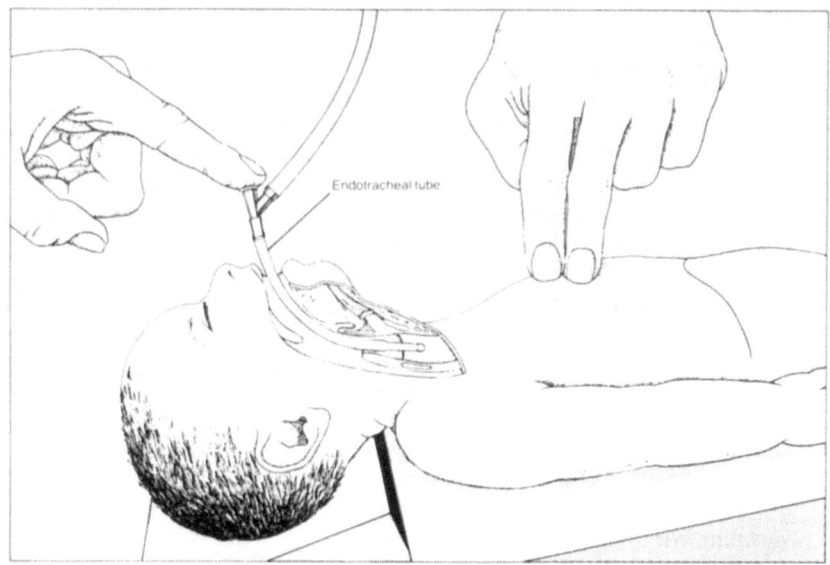

Figure 11   *External cardiac massage with two fingers on the midsternum*

an association between sodium bicarbonate therapy and intraventricular haemorrhage in preterm infants. If used, a dose of 1–2 mmol/kg of 8.4% sodium bicarbonate should be given through an umbilical venous catheter. It should be diluted with an equal volume of water and given slowly over two to five minutes. If the bradycardia still persists this can be followed by adrenaline, calcium chloride and dextrose given intravenously (Table 7).

Table 7   Drug therapy

Drug	Concentration	Indication	Route	Dose
Sodium bicarbonate	8.4% (1 mmol/ml)	Metabolic acidosis	i.v.	1–2 mmol/kg (diluted)
Adrenaline	1:10 000	Asystole	i.v.	0.1 ml/kg
Calcium chloride	10%	Low cardiac output	i.v.	0.1 ml/kg
Dextrose	20%	Hypoglycaemia	i.v.	1 ml/kg
Naloxone	0.02 mg/ml (neonatal)	Pethidine within four hours	i.v. or i.m.	0.01 mg/kg

Shock

Some infants are shocked following severe intrapartum blood loss. They are pale, tachypnoeic, tachycardic and hypotensive with weak pulses. Group O rhesus negative blood or a plasma expander should be given immediately via an umbilical venous catheter, at a rate of 20 ml/kg over 30 minutes. Infants may also be in shock from persistent severe acidosis.

Maternal analgesia

If the mother has received pethidine within four hours of delivery, the infant's respiratory drive may be depressed. These babies are usually easy to oxygenate and the heart rate responds rapidly but they make poor respiratory effort. The infant should be ventilated and a morphine antagonist, naloxone, given, either intravenously via a peripheral vein, or more conveniently and safely by intramuscular injection. It takes a few minutes for the drug to take effect if given intramuscularly, and ventilation can be supported during this time. Naloxone does not cause respiratory depression but its effect is short-lived and it may need to be repeated. There is no place for respiratory stimulants in neonates.

Meconium aspiration

The aspiration of thick, 'pea soup' meconium can result in severe postnatal anoxia, and death. When thick particulate meconium is present, the infant's mouth should be sucked out with a mucus extractor or large calibre suction catheter immediately the baby's head appears. This reduces the incidence of meconium aspiration. As soon as the child is placed on the resuscitaire, suction under direct vision should be performed. The infant should be intubated with as large an endotracheal tube as possible, and the meconium aspirated by sucking on the end of the endotracheal tube while withdrawing it. Speed is needed to try and suck out the meconium before the infant's first gasp. Putting a piece of gauze or a face mask over the end of the tube will prevent getting a mouthful of meconium. This procedure should be repeated until no more meconium is aspirated, but without allowing significant bradycardia to occur. A fine suction catheter passed down the inside of the endotracheal tube will not remove the meconium successfully.

Hypothermia

Babies should not be allowed to become hypothermic. Resuscitation should be performed under a radiant heater, and the baby dried promptly and wrapped in a warm towel as soon as resuscitation has been completed.

Preterm infants

It is particularly important not to allow infants whose gestational age is less than thirty-two weeks to become hypoxic, and prompt and efficient resuscitation with early intubation and a period of intermittent positive pressure ventilation is often required to achieve this. Acute hypoxia will be accompanied by hypercapnia and surges in blood pressure, and all these have been implicated as major factors in the pathogenesis of intraventricular haemorrhages (Pape and Wigglesworth, 1979) which is the major cause of death in infants of this gestation. Adequate ventilation is also important for the release of surfactant from pneumocytes, and every effort should be made to prevent hypoxia, acidaemia and hypothermia as they will all adversely affect surfactant synthesis.

Preterm infants are particularly prone to becoming hypothermic. To prevent this, in addition to the measures already described, the delivery room should be as warm as possible, and during resuscitation the baby can be covered with a sheet of bubble plastic. This is preferable to wrapping the baby in a towel as it still allows easy access and visibility. The preterm infant should be transferred without any unnecessary delay to a warm portable incubator. If indicated, the endotracheal tube may be left *in situ*, secured and attached to the portable ventilator before transferring the baby to the neonatal unit.

Caesarean section

Following delivery by Caesarean section with the mother under a general anaesthetic, it is not uncommon for babies to cry initially, and then become apnoeic. Many of these babies need to be intubated and given intermittent positive pressure ventilation. Lung liquid may be seen welling up the trachea, and needs to be sucked out to be able to visualize the vocal cords.

Stopping resuscitation

Resuscitation should be instituted whenever a heart rate has been recorded or heard during the second stage of labour even if no heart rate is present at birth. In a series of infants where no heart sounds at all could be detected at birth some survived without handicap (Scott 1976).

If there is no effective cardiac output or spontaneous respiration after 30 minutes of resuscitation, further efforts are usually unrewarding. Where a cardiac output is obtained but no spontaneous respiration established, the infant should be put on a portable ventilator and transferred to the neonatal unit for further evaluation.

Parents

Most infants respond rapidly to resuscitation even when intubation is required. After rapid examination the infant should be wrapped up and handed to the mother to hold. It should be explained to the parents that their child has required assistance to start breathing but they can be reassured that the prognosis is excellent. Even if the baby has to be transferred to the neonatal unit it is important for the mother to hold her baby, or, if ventilation is required, to be able to see and stroke him in the portable incubator before he is transferred.

References

Apgar, V. (1953), *Curr. Res. Anesth. Analg.*, **32**, 260.

Dawes, G. S. (1968), *Foetal and Neonatal Physiology*, Year Book Publishers, London and Chicago.

Pape, K. E. and Wigglesworth, J. S. (1979), *Haemorrhage, Ischaemia and the Perinatal Brain*. Spastics International Medical Publications. Heinemann, London.

Scott, H. (1976), *Arch. Dis. Child.*, **51**, 712

Further reading

Davenport, H. T. and Valman, H. B. (1980), Resuscitation of the newborn in *General Anaesthesia*, Vol. 2, Cecil Gray, T., Nunn, J. F. and Utting, J. E. (Eds.), Butterworths, London.

Gregory, G. A. (1975), Resuscitation of the newborn. *Anesthesiology*, **43**, 2, 225.

Hull, D. (1971), Asphyxia neonatorum in *Recent Advances in Paediatrics*, Gairdner, D. and Hull, D. (Eds.), Churchill Livingstone, Edinburgh.

CHAPTER 2

Cardiorespiratory arrest

The principles of management of cardiorespiratory arrest in children and adults are the same but important differences exist. These arise from the differences in anatomy and physiology between children and adults and from the adjustments which need to be made to techniques of resuscitation and doses of drugs.

Most cardiac arrests in children are preceded by respiratory insufficiency. Children with respiratory distress, and those at risk of hypoxia, need to be closely observed and monitored. In addition, some cardiac arrests may be prevented by the early recognition and correction of hypoglycaemia, electrolyte abnormalities, shock and septicaemia.

The earlier effective resuscitation is instituted, the better the prognosis. In adults who have not been hypoxic prior to cardiorespiratory arrest, there appears to be a period of about four minutes before discernible brain damage occurs (Cole and Corday, 1956). In children hypoxia usually precedes cardiac arrest and the critical time interval is likely to be shorter.

Resuscitation

Resuscitation should be instituted immediately the diagnosis is made and irrespective of the place where the cardiorespiratory arrest occurs. The most important aspects—establishing an airway, breathing for the patient and re-establishing the circulation by external

21

cardiac massage—can be done single-handed and without any equipment. It is only by the rapid initiation of these measures that a successful outcome may be achieved. If there is any doubt about the diagnosis, it is best to assume that a cardiorespiratory arrest has occurred and start resuscitation.

In hospital there should be a well-established, simple procedure for immediately summoning the members of staff and equipment needed to assist in the resuscitation. Rapid and orderly team work is required under the direction of the most senior doctor present or a previously designated leader. In addition, the time, sequence of events and drugs given should be recorded during the resuscitation.

Resuscitation equipment specifically designed for children must be available in the accident and emergency department and on the children's wards. Figure 1 shows how such equipment can be con-

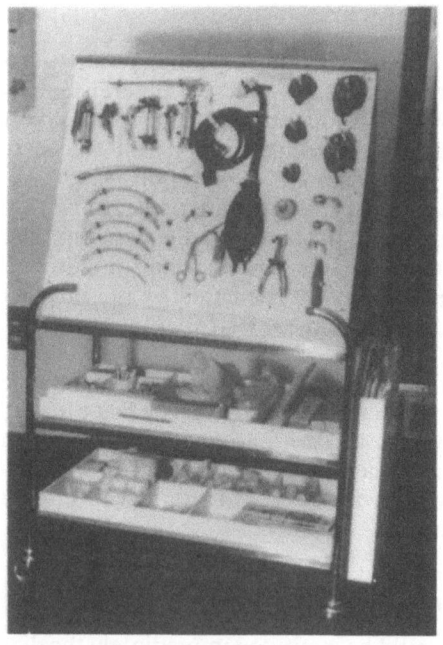

Figure 1   *Equipment needed for cardiorespiratory arrest displayed on a mobile board. Beneath each item is a photograph of it, allowing any missing items to be readily identified*

veniently displayed on a mobile board and trolley, so that the item required can be instantly recognized.

The same orderly sequence for the conduct of cardiopulmonary arrest as listed in the mnemonic ABCDEF (airway, breathing, circulation, drugs, ECG, fluids and follow-up) applies equally well to children as to adults (Figure 2).

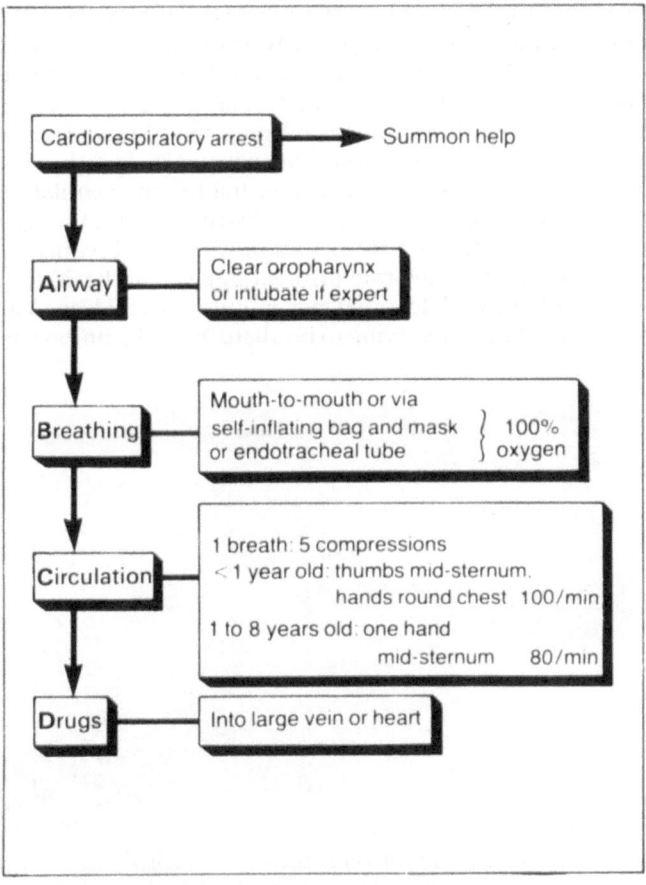

Figure 2 *Management of cardiorespiratory arrest*

A for airway and B for breathing

The airway must be cleared of vomit and secretions, either manually or, preferably, by mechanical suction. Artificial respiration must then begin using either the mouth-to-mouth method, or, preferably, a self-inflating bag and mask attached to 100% oxygen. An oral airway should first be inserted. Almost all children can be adequately ventilated with a self-inflating bag and mask; care should be taken to ensure that the seal between the face and mask is adequate and not to over-extend the head as this will occlude the airway. The mandible should not be pulled up too vigorously as this may cause the tongue to press against the soft palate and occlude the nasopharynx (Figure 3). In neonates, the mouth-to-mouth technique has to be modified to cover both the mouth and nose and only mouthfuls of air are required. Movement of the chest wall with each breath will show whether or not ventilation is adequate. Inadequate ventilation may be the result of improper technique or obstruction by a foreign body. It is recommended to start resuscitation with four breaths in rapid succession. Thereafter, the rate of breathing should be 20 times per minute for infants and 15 times per minute for children. Valuable time should not be lost by trying to intubate the child, unless someone

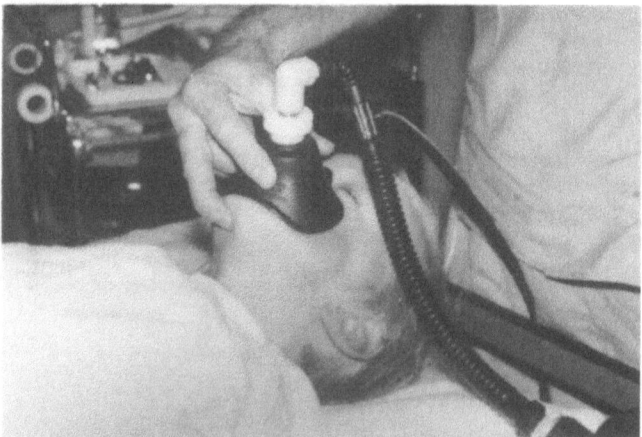

Figure 3 *Demonstration of correct position for holding the head when ventilating a child with a self-inflating bag and mask. Here the mask is attached to an anaesthetic circuit, but this should be used only by anaesthetists*

24

competent in this skill is present, when an endotracheal tube should be passed. An uncuffed endotracheal tube should be used, and its diameter (Table 1) corresponds approximately to the diameter of the patient's little finger or can be calculated from the formula:

$$\frac{age}{4} + 4 = \text{internal diameter (mm)}$$

Table 1   Sizes of endotracheal tubes

Age	Internal diameter (mm)	French gauge	Length (cm)
1-6 months	3.5	14-16	10
12-18 months	4.0	18-20	12
3-4 years	5.0	22-24	14
7-9 years	6.0	26-28	16

A nasogastric tube should be passed to prevent abdominal distension.

C for circulation

External cardiac massage is used to re-establish the circulation. In adults an initial precordial thump on the chest is recommended in certain circumstances. In children, however, it is rarely successful, is more likely to cause damage, and should not be done.

For infants less than one year old, cardiac massage is best performed by encircling the chest with both hands and exerting pressure with both thumbs over the midsternum (Figure 4). For older children, cardiac massage can be performed with the heel of one hand placed on the midsternum. The heart lies relatively higher in the thorax in children and exerting pressure over the lower sternum is less effective and may cause rupture of the liver. Cardiac massage is performed most effectively on a hard surface, so that the heart can be compressed firmly between the sternum and the spine. Complete relaxation must be ensured between compressions to allow the heart to fill. The adequacy of massage must be monitored at regular intervals by palpation of the femoral or brachial pulses. The carotid pulse may be difficult to feel in infants because of their short and often fat necks. The rhythm is one breath alternating with five compressions

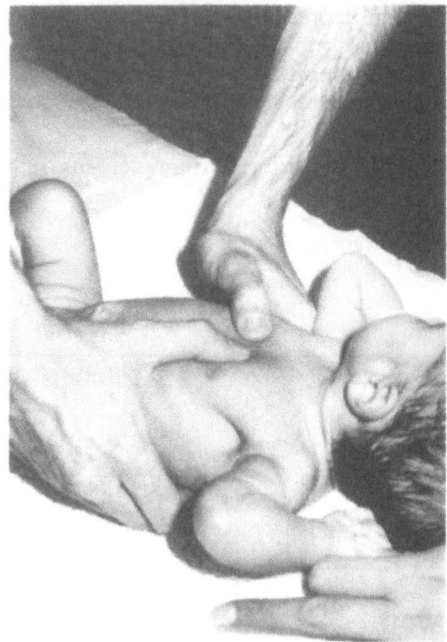

Figure 4 *External cardiac massage in an infant, performed with both hands on the midsternum and the hands encircling the chest*

of the chest, aiming to maintain a pulse rate of 100 per minute in infants and 80 per minute in children, and can be established by counting. In an infant one counts one, two, three, four, five, breathe; in a child one and two and three and four and five and breathe.

D for drugs

Once adequate respiration and circulation have been established, an intravenous line should be inserted in as central a vessel as possible. If this proves difficult, a cut down can be performed on the long saphenous vein or a vein in the antecubital fossa but it is usually quicker to start a drip percutaneously. In infants a scalp vein can be used. In desperate circumstances boluses of drugs can be given into the heart. A FG 20 needle can either be inserted in the angle between the xiphisternum and the rib cage and directed upwards and posteriorly, or in the fourth intercostal space on the left, just medial and below the left nipple, aiming towards the spine. When hypovolaemia has been the cause of the arrest, appropriate fluid replacement with a plasma expander should be given. Fluid therapy will also be required to counteract the hypovolaemia from capillary leakage following hypoxia. A guide to drug therapy is shown in Figure 5 and Table 2 lists appropriate drug doses.

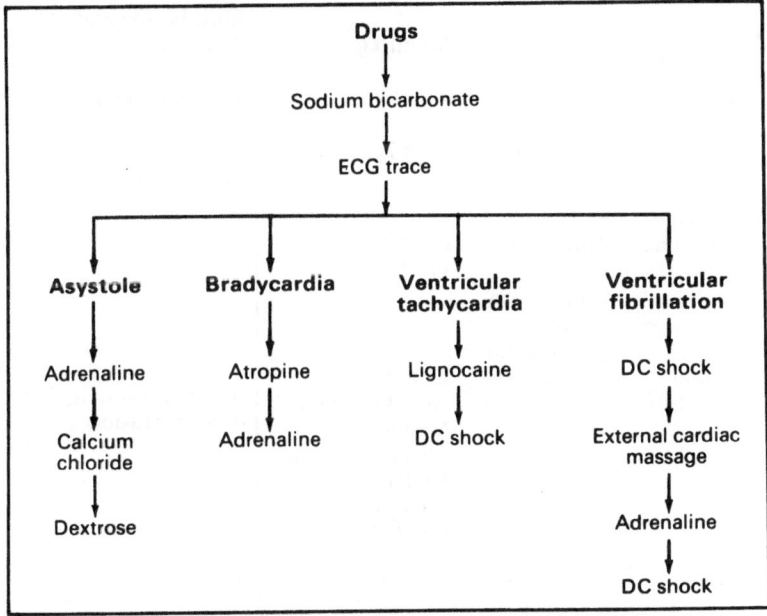

Figure 5   *Drugs used in the management of cardiac arrest*

Correction of acidosis

It has been traditional to treat vigorously the acidosis which follows a cardiac arrest. Very severe acidosis will adversely affect cardiovascular function, and the drugs which stimulate cardiac contractility are not effective in the presence of a profound acidosis, making restoration of normal cardiac function more difficult. It is now clear that a major component of the acidosis, the respiratory acidosis, can

Table 2 Appropriate drug doses for cardiorespiratory arrest in children. Use the 'rule of ones' for bolus doses

Drug	Concentration	Dose	Indication
Bolus doses, given intravenously or intracardiac			
Adrenaline	1 : 10 000	0.1 ml/kg	Asystole, bradycardia, ventricular fibrillation
Atropine	0.6 mg/ml	0.01 mg/kg	Sinus bradycardia, AV block
Bicarbonate	8.4%	1 ml/kg	Acidosis—ventilation must be adequate
Calcium chloride	10%	0.1 ml/kg	Asystole
Dextrose	20%	1 ml/kg	Hypoglycaemia in infants
Lignocaine	2% (20 mg/ml)	1 mg/kg	Ventricular tachycardia
Infusion doses			
Isoprenaline	2 mg/2 ml	$0.1-0.5\,\mu g$ $kg^{-1}\,min^{-1}$	
	Mix 2 mg in 500 ml to give 4 μg/ml		
Dopamine	200 mg/5 ml	Low dose: $5\,\mu g\,kg^{-1}\,min^{-1}$ Medium dose: $10\,\mu g\,kg^{-1}\,min^{-1}$ High dose: $20\,\mu g\,kg^{-1}\,min^{-1}$ (see Table 3 for details)	Electrical activity but poor perfusion

be managed by ensuring adequate alveolar ventilation without using sodium bicarbonate. Attention has also recently been focused on the possible hazards of giving large doses of sodium bicarbonate, particularly as it may cause a paradoxical worsening of the acidosis in the central nervous system rather than improving it. There is also the added risk of giving a hyperosmolar solution with a high concentration of sodium. A compromise is to give 1 mmol/kg (1 ml/kg of 8.4%) sodium bicarbonate initially if hypoxia has been prolonged and then treat the acidosis according to blood gas results. The dose of further sodium bicarbonate (mmol/l) can be calculated from the formula:

Base deficit (mmol/l) × 0.3 × weight (kg)

The sodium bicarbonate will be helpful only if effective ventilation has been established to remove excess carbon dioxide.

E for ECG tracing

The ECG is needed to determine subsequent drug therapy. If no ECG trace is available, it can be assumed that the child is in asystole, as this is usually the case.

Asystole

Adrenaline (epinephrine). The beneficial effects of adrenaline have been well substantiated. It elevates the perfusion pressure generated during cardiac compression, improves myocardial contractility, stimulates spontaneous contractions and may convert fine ventricular fibrillation to coarse ventricular fibrillation which is more responsive to defibrillation. Only the 1 in 10 000 strength solution should be used, preferably intravenously. If an infusion cannot be rapidly established, a similar dose can be instilled down the endotracheal tube into the tracheobronchial tree (Roberts *et al.*, 1979).

Calcium. The calcium ion increases myocardial contractility and it may enhance ventricular excitability. It may be useful in electro-mechanical dissocation where there is organized electrical activity but ineffective myocardial contraction, and in some cases of ventricular standstill. It should be given slowly and preferably not via the intracardiac route, as intramyocardial injection may produce necrosis. It is recommended to give the calcium as calcium chloride, as it is already in the ionized form and available directly to the tissues.

Dextrose. In infants there may be accompanying hypoglycaemia. This can be rapidly checked with a Dextrostix or BM-Test-Glycemie '20-800' strip, and dextrose given if necessary.

If no effect is obtained from giving these drugs, additional sodium bicarbonate may be required, and a further dose of each drug given. If all these are ineffective, intracardiac adrenaline or intravenous isoprenaline can be tried.

Inotropic agents

When there is satisfactory electrical activity of the heart but hypotension and poor perfusion, inotropic agents may be helpful.

Isoprenaline (isoproterenol). This stimulates β-adrenergic receptors. It improves cardiac output by increasing both the heart rate and the force of myocardial contraction and there is peripheral arterial dilatation particularly in skeletal muscle. Myocardial oxygen consumption is also increased. It is also a patent bronchodilator. As it is a powerful inotropic agent, the increase in cardiac output will usually compensate for the decreased peripheral resistance. Care needs to be taken to ensure that the patient is normovolaemic, and that an adequate central venous pressure is maintained during therapy. Although the net effect of isoprenaline is to increase systemic blood flow, a disproportionate amount may go to skeletal muscle at the expense of the renal blood flow and urine output may diminish. This may be overcome by the simultaneous infusion of a low dose of dopamine. It often produces a marked tachycardia, and initially a low dose is used and titrated with the response. Isoprenaline can be used in shock when the blood pressure is low and cardiac output is deteriorating, and for bradycardia which has not responded to atropine.

Dopamine. Dopamine has both α- and β-receptor stimulating actions. Its effects differ with the dose given and individual response differs with a given dose. In low dosage it increases renal, mesenteric and coronary arterial blood flow, with either a slight decrease or no change in the peripheral vascular resistance. When the dose is increased, it has a β-stimulatory effect on the heart with increased myocardial contractility and cardiac output. In high dosage, there is

Table 3 Dopamine infusion regime: use 200 mg (5 ml) dopamine in 500 ml of 5% dextrose, to give 400 μg/ml

Weight (kg)	Infusion rate (ml/h)		
	Low dose	Medium dose	High dose
5	4	8	15
10	8	15	30
20	15	30	60
50	30	75	150

an α-receptor stimulating effect, with peripheral vasoconstriction. Starting with a low dose, the strength of the infusion is gradually increased according to the response in blood pressure and renal output (Table 3). It should not be discontinued abruptly, and is inactivated by sodium bicarbonate. It is mainly used to improve perfusion in low cardiac output states after hypovolaemia has been corrected.

Dobutamine. This is a synthetic β-receptor stimulant. It increases myocardial contractility with minimal peripheral vasoconstriction. Unlike dopamine it does not specifically increase renal and mesenteric blood flow. It may be used in the treatment of shock where there is inadequate myocardial contractility.

Adrenaline. This can also be given by low dose continuous infusion to improve cardiac output and hypotension in shock. It should be given into a central vein and may cause severe vasoconstriction.

Whenever any of these agents is given, the patient must have close monitoring of central venous pressure, ECG, blood pressure and urine output. All these drugs can cause cardiac arrhythmias. The preference for particular agents varies between different units, but isoprenaline is the most widely used inotropic agent in children, and can be combined with dopamine in low dose to augment renal blood flow.

Ventricular fibrillation

In cases of ventricular fibrillation, which is particularly likely after an electric shock, electric defibrillation should be given. An example of a portable defibrillator with a paddle attachment for a child is shown in Figure 6. The largest electrode paddle that allows good chest contact over its entire area should be used. Electrode jelly is applied to the paddles and one is placed to the right of the sternum and the other over the apex of the heart. Warn everybody to stand clear of the bed before giving the shock. A suitable setting for the initial DC shock is 10 J/year or 2 J/kg (Gutgesell *et al.*, 1976). Cardiac massage should begin again immediately after defibrillation. If the initial shock is unsuccessful, adrenaline can also be given followed by a further shock at double the energy. Defibrillation is unlikely to be successful in the presence of severe acidosis.

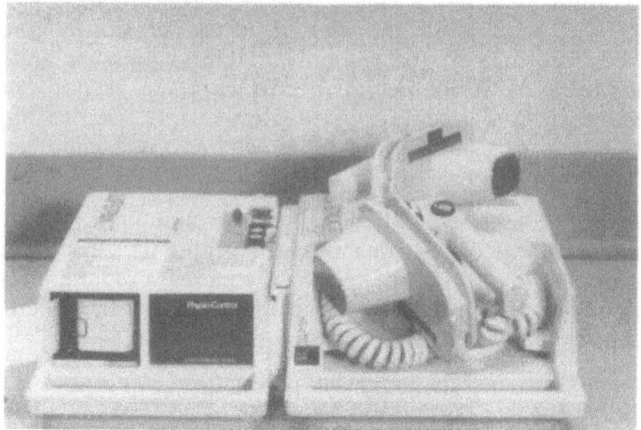

Figure 6   *Portable defibrillator with paddle attachments for a child*

F for follow-up

The most important single prognostic indicator is the duration and degree of anoxia sustained.

Following successful resuscitation, the child should be transferred to the intensive care unit. In addition to the many supportive measures and monitoring required for such a child, attention is increasingly being directed towards the prevention of postanoxic cerebral oedema. In addition, intravenous barbiturates given in very high doses have recently been used to reduce the cerebral metabolic rate and enhance the utilization of oxygen and glucose. Some of the measures available are described in more detail in the chapter on coma (Chapter 10).

If resuscitation is unsuccessful, the most senior doctor will have to decide when to abandon the procedure. This decision is seldom easy, but if there is no cardiovascular responsiveness after 30 minutes of effective resuscitation, further attempts are almost always unrewarding. Exceptions to this may be drug overdose and cold water drowning. Following drowning in extremely cold water, isolated cases have been recorded of asystole lasting several hours before the return of any vital signs, yet with good neurological recovery.

References

Cole, S. and Corday, E. (1956), *J. Am. Med. Assoc.*, **161,** 1454.
Gutgesell, H. P., Tacker, W. A., Geddes, L. A., Davis, J. S., Lie, J. T. and McNamara, D. G. (1976), *Pediatrics*, **58,** 898.
Roberts, J. R., Greenberg, M. I., Knaub, M. A. (1979), *JACEP*, **8,** 515.

Further reading

Driscoll, D., Gillette, P. and McNamara, D. (1978), The use of dopamine in children, *J. Pediatr.*, **92,** 309.
Standards and Guidelines for Cardiopulmonary Resuscitation (CPR) and Emergency Cardiac Care (ECC) (1980), *J. Am. Med. Assoc.*, **244,** 453. This is an extensive and authoritative account of cardiorespiratory resuscitation in both adults and children.

CHAPTER 3

The child with stridor

Acute stridor in a child is an alarming experience for everyone concerned. The child is frightened by his difficulty in breathing, the parent by the noise and distress it is causing and the doctor by his appreciation of the potential gravity of the situation. This chapter describes some of the main causes of acute stridor and their management.

Definition

Stridor is the harsh sound caused by the presence of an obstruction to breathing in the larynx or trachea. It is derived from 'stridulus'

Table 1   Causes of stridor

Acute	*Chronic*
Laryngotracheobronchitis	Congenital laryngeal stridor
Epiglottitis	Foreign body
Foreign body	Vocal cord paralysis
Retropharyngeal abscess	Vascular ring
Post-intubation	Subglottic stenosis
Diphtheria	Micrognathia
Angio-oedema	Laryngeal lesions
Hypocalcaemia	—congenital laryngeal webs
Steam or smoke inhalation injury	—cysts, papillomata
	Tracheal lesions
	—subglottic haemangioma

meaning whistling or grating. The timing of the stridor can be helpful. If it is mainly inspiratory it suggests an extrathoracic airway obstruction; if there is an expiratory component the obstruction involves the intrathoracic airways. It needs to be contrasted with wheezing, which is higher pitched and is a prolonged expiratory sound produced by intrathoracic airways obstruction. They may co-exist, and parents may think that their child is wheezing when he actually has stridor.

The causes of stridor can be divided into acute and chronic, and are shown in Table 1.

Laryngotracheobronchitis

This is by far the most common cause of stridor in children. It is often called 'croup' but care needs to be taken with this term as it is sometimes used to describe stridor of any origin.

Laryngotracheobronchitis is almost always viral in origin. Para-influenza virus type 1 is the organism most commonly isolated, although para-influenza types 2 and 3, respiratory syncytial virus and influenza viruses are also found. Measles is occasionally a cause. In half the cases presenting no virus can be isolated. Most cases occur between October and March when at least one of these viruses is prevalent in the community.

The larynx, trachea, bronchi and indeed any part of the respiratory tract may be affected. Although there may be widespread inflammatory oedema of the respiratory mucosa and submucosa, the site which causes the major symptoms is the subglottic area. The supraglottic area is relatively unaffected.

Clinical features

The majority of patients are between six months and three years of age. Preceding symptoms of an upper respiratory tract infection are common. These are followed by a harsh barking cough with a hoarse voice—the most characteristic features of the illness. A low-grade fever is often present and the stridor frequently starts or is worse at night. When mild, the stridor is predominantly inspiratory, harsh and easily audible. If the disease progresses there will be supraclavicular and substernal recession and the stridor may become both inspiratory and expiratory. There may also be a wheeze associated with involvement of the smaller airways.

With severe disease there are two main problems, respiratory obstruction and hypoxia. Hypoxia causes tachypnoea, tachycardia, restlessness and eventually cyanosis. With increasing respiratory obstruction, the child will have increasing chest recession and stridor and eventually exhaustion may follow, which may be accompanied by a decrease in the recession and a quietening of the stridor. This may be falsely attributed to an improvement in the clinical condition of the child, but is caused by a reduction in airflow, detectable by careful examination of the chest for adequacy of air entry. A sudden reduction in stridor and recession may be an ominous rather than a good sign.

In most cases the signs of respiratory obstruction abate in a day or two, although the cough lasts up to a week. Many children have recurrent episodes, with successive viral upper respiratory tract infections.

Diagnosis

The diagnosis is usually made on the history and clinical findings, but other causes of stridor, in particular acute epiglottitis and an inhaled foreign body, need to be considered in all cases. The place of radiographs is controversial, but if there is any doubt about the

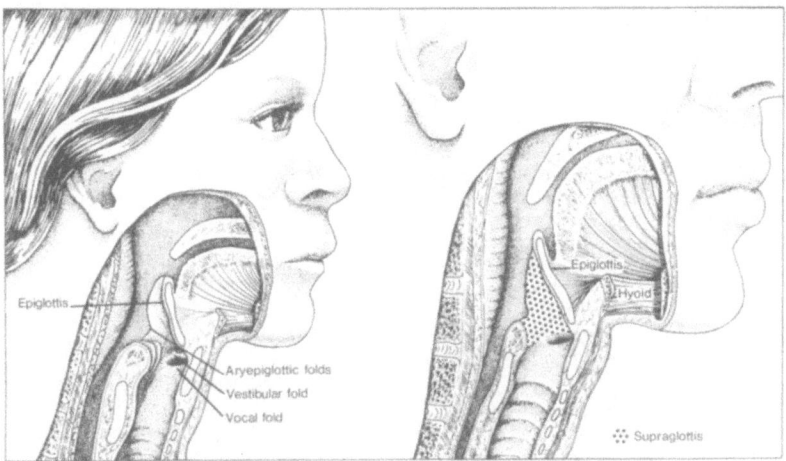

Figure 1   *Anatomy of the neck showing the supraglottis*

diagnosis, or if the illness is severe enough to require hospital admission, a lateral radiograph of the neck and a chest radiograph which includes the upper airway can be very helpful. It may enable one to confirm the diagnosis and exclude an inhaled foreign body, epiglottitis and a retropharyngeal abscess. The normal anatomy of the larynx and trachea is shown in Figure 1, and the normal appearance of the airways on a lateral radiograph of the neck is shown in Figure 2a. The subglottic narrowing seen in laryngotracheobronchitis is shown in Figure 2b, and the features of epiglottitis in Figure 2c.

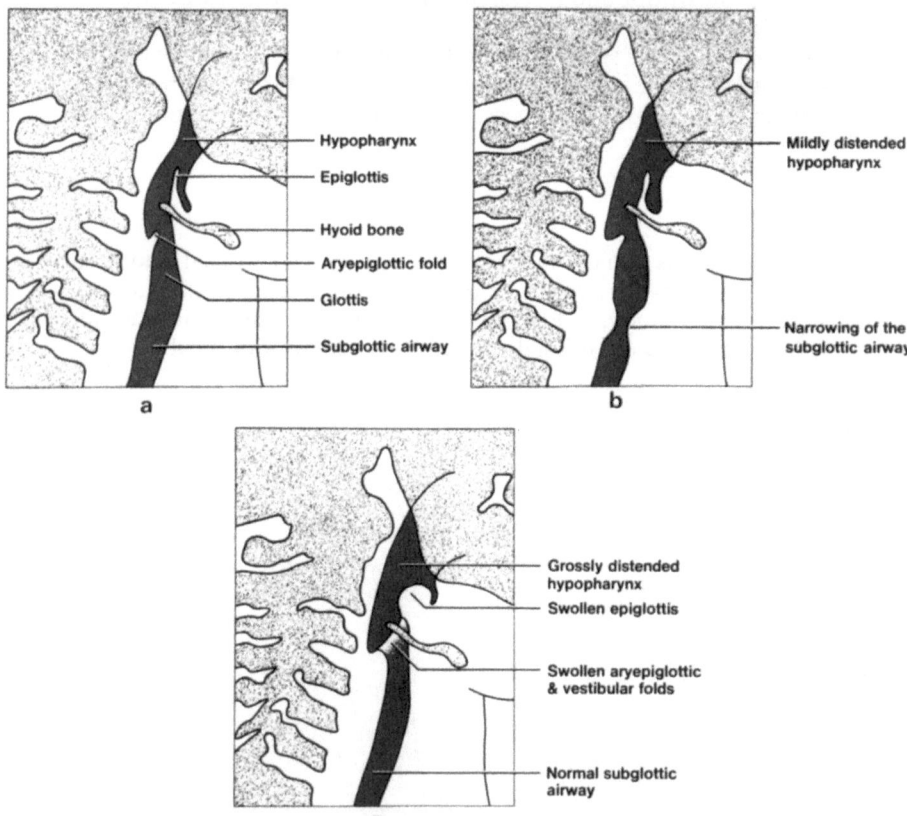

Figure 2   *Diagrammatic representation of the lateral neck*
(a) *Normal* **(b)** *Laryngotracheobronchitis* **(c)** *Epiglottitis*

Home or hospital?

Most children have mild disease and are managed at home, the usual advice being to nurse them in a humid environment. This can be achieved by taking the child into the bathroom and turning on the hot water tap, or with a humidifier.

In the casualty department it may be difficult to assess the severity of the disease, and the decision to admit or discharge may not be easy. A child with marked stridor and recession, particularly when not crying, should be admitted. Any child with signs of hypoxia will certainly need admission. A markedly raised respiratory rate, restlessness, altered state of consciousness or cyanosis all suggest hypoxia. It is also advisable to admit most infants under one year old. Children who are less ill but whose parents are having difficulty coping, or where there are adverse home conditions, may need brief admission.

Hospital treatment

Children with laryngotracheobronchitis are anxious and distressed. Their ventilation will be compromised if they are crying or upset. They should be disturbed as little as possible, but not to the exclusion of careful observation. Unpleasant investigations should be avoided, in particular examination of the throat with a spatula is contraindicated, as it may precipitate respiratory obstruction.

Most of these children are nursed in a transparent tent or 'croupette' (Figure 3). The use of mist in the tent is traditional and does appear to give symptomatic relief. The main disadvantages of these tents are that they make observation much more difficult and many children find them frightening. Good hydration is important and can usually be managed orally. Frequent observation is vital in order to detect the onset of respiratory failure.

Intubation

Respiratory obstruction needing intubation is an uncommon complication of laryngotracheobronchitis. Only about 3% of children admitted to hospital will have such severe disease, but as laryngotracheobronchitis is a relatively common illness, this is not an insignificant number and children still die from this disease if they are not managed appropriately.

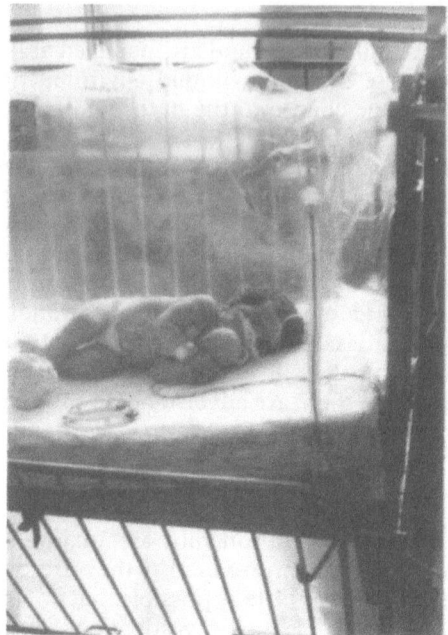

Figure 3 *A 20-month-old child in a tent receiving humidified oxygen, and playing with toys. He required intubation for laryngotracheobronchitis and has a nasotracheal and nasogastric tube*

The need for intubation is dictated by the severity of the subglottic obstruction and whether or not the child is hypoxic in spite of treatment. The severity of subglottic obstruction correlates with the degree of stridor and chest recession, whereas the best clinical guide to hypoxia is the respiratory rate and tachycardia. Irritability and restlessness are later signs, and any impairment of consciousness or cyanosis are indications for urgent intervention. Intubation may also be required if the child's condition deteriorates suddenly if secretions cause airways obstruction.

Respiratory failure

If the child is in marked respiratory difficulty, or any signs of severe hypoxia are present, immediate relief of the airway obstruction is

40

required. Children who are deteriorating more slowly should have their blood gases measured. Hypoxia in spite of oxygen, a steadily rising Pa_{CO_2} or a Pa_{CO_2} greater than 7 kPa (53 mmHg) indicate the need for intervention.

In most cases a nasotracheal tube is used (Figure 4), and the appropriate size is shown in Table 2. Smaller tubes than normal are

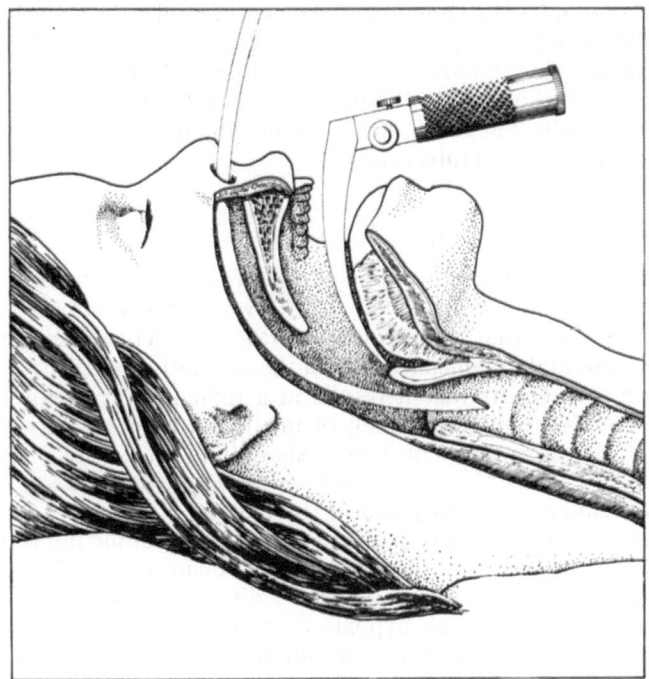

Figure 4   *Nasotracheal tube in place*

Table 2   **Size of nasotracheal tube used in children with laryngotracheo-bronchitis and epiglottitis**

Age	Size
6 months–3 years	3·5 mm
3–5 years	4·0 mm
> 5 years	4·5 mm

used to negotiate the obstruction and to avoid trauma. Intubation should preferably be performed by an anaesthetist skilled in paediatrics and facilities for an immediate tracheostomy must be available in case intubation is not possible or does not bypass completely the tracheal narrowing. Intubation is preferable to tracheostomy as it can be done more rapidly and easily, no surgery is required, and the postoperative complications of a tracheostomy are avoided. The children are nursed in humidified oxygen, the tube is regularly suctioned with saline and physiotherapy is performed. The nasotracheal tube can usually be removed after two to five days, when the subglottic oedema has resolved sufficiently to enable the child to breathe around the tube. Subglottic stenosis following removal of the tube is uncommon if a small tube is used.

Other treatments

In North America racemic epinephrine (a mixture of the D- and L-isomers of adrenaline) is widely used, given as a nebulized aerosol. The rationale is that it has a topical vasoconstrictive effect on the oedematous and inflamed mucosa of the subglottic area. There have been several reports that it results in a reduction in the need for intubation. It should be used only on inpatients, as it causes a marked tachycardia and its benefit is only short lived. It is rarely used in Britain.

Ipecacuanha has been given in the past as it appears to reduce laryngeal spasm, but it may induce vomiting and should not be used. The use of steroids is controversial, there being no conclusive evidence that they alter the course of the disease. Sedation is contraindicated as it may mask hypoxia or even produce it by reducing respiratory drive. Antibiotics are not routinely used as secondary bacterial infection is rare.

Acute epiglottitis

Acute epiglottitis is rarer than laryngotracheobronchitis, but the diagnosis must be considered in all children with stridor or respiratory distress. The epiglottis may be grossly swollen and cherry-red from inflammation and oedema. However, swelling of the surrounding structures, particularly the aryepiglottic folds, may be more important and 'supraglottitis' would be a more appropriate name. It usually occurs in children from three to seven years and carries a high mortality. Sudden death may result from respiratory obstruction after the child has been ill for only a few hours, so any delay in making the diagnosis or initiating treatment may be disastrous. It is worth bearing in mind that many of the early cases of epiglottitis described in England were reported by pathologists from postmortem findings. If children presenting at hospital with epiglottitis are to survive, a well-organized plan of action is crucial.

Almost all cases are caused by group B *Haemophilus influenzae*. Septicaemia occurs in most cases of epiglottitis, but spread to distant foci causing meningitis or septic arthritis is extremely rare.

Clinical features

Epiglottitis is an illness of sudden onset, although about a quarter of cases may have had a preceding upper respiratory tract infection. A severe sore throat develops abruptly, accompanied by a high temperature. The illness progresses rapidly, with severe dysphagia which often prevents swallowing of saliva, resulting in dribbling. The voice is muffled but unlike laryngotracheobronchitis coughing is not a feature. Respiratory distress is present in most cases, with supraclavicular and substernal recession, and although stridor is usually present it is often quiet and not a prominent feature.

The appearance of the child with epiglottitis is very characteristic. He looks ill, sits upright and leans forward with his chin up and mouth open to create the optimal airway, and saliva dribbles down the front of his mouth. These classical features are not always present, but drooling from difficulty in swallowing is usually a clue to the diagnosis. A comparison of the clinical features of laryngotracheobronchitis and epiglottitis are shown in Table 3.

Management

All cases must be admitted and need urgent attention. A paediatrician and an anaesthetist should be called immediately, and resuscitation equipment made available, as complete airways obstruction may occur at any time. The throat should never be examined, the child should not be disturbed or efforts made to make him lie down, as any of these may precipitate a respiratory arrest. All these children should be taken straight to the intensive care unit or operating

Table 3 Differences between laryngotracheobronchitis and epiglottitis

	Laryngotracheobronchitis	*Epiglottitis*
Clinical Features		
Causative organism	Para-influenza virus	*Haemophilus influenzae*
Peak age	6 months–3 years	3–7 years
Preceding URTI	Usual	Less common
Onset	Days	Hours
Sore throat	Unusual	Severe
Dysphagia	Absent	Severe, dribbling
Voice	Hoarse with barking cough	Muffled
Clinical state	Mildly unwell	Toxic and ill
Temperature	None or slight	High
Stridor	Marked	Soft
Posture	No preference	Sitting and leaning forward
Investigations		
WBC	Unremarkable	Marked neutrophilia
Blood culture	Negative	Positive for *Haemophilus influenzae*
Lateral neck radiograph	Normal epiglottis, subglottic narrowing	Swollen epiglottis and aryepiglottic folds, distended hypopharynx
Management		
	Humidity ± oxygen	Chloramphenicol ± ampicillin
	Occasional intubation	Intubation in most cases

theatre. At all times the child must be accompanied by a member of the medical staff who would be able to intubate and resuscitate the child if necessary. The place of lateral neck radiographs continues to be debated. For good quality radiographs, the neck needs to be extended and this may precipitate respiratory obstruction, although this is very rare. If the child is very ill and the clinical features suggest epiglottitis, taking radiographs is contra-indicated, as they are unnecessary, waste valuable time, and are potentially hazardous. When the diagnosis is not clearcut, lateral neck radiographs can be very useful, and may prevent milder or atypical cases from being missed. The radiographic appearance in epiglottitis is shown in Figure 5.

Early intervention to guarantee an airway is preferable to waiting

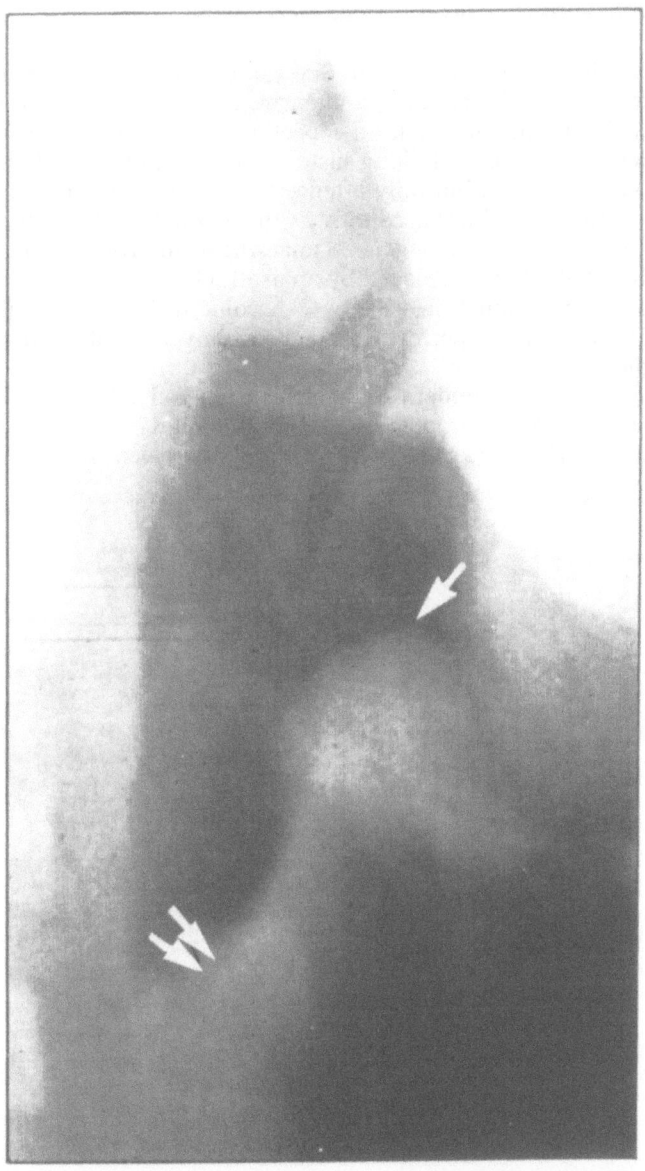

Figure 5 *Lateral neck radiograph in acute epiglottitis showing the characteristic features. The epiglottis is swollen and thumb shaped (✝), the aryepiglottic folds are widened (✝✝), and the hypopharynx is distended*

for a respiratory arrest to occur. Several trials have shown that even children closely observed in an intensive care unit may die or suffer irreversible brain damage if an expectant policy is followed. A few children with a relatively long history who are not very ill may be cautiously observed but only after very careful evaluation. Intubation has superseded tracheostomy as the method of choice to guarantee the airway. Under a general anaesthetic an orotracheal tube is passed initially but is replaced by a nasotracheal tube shortly afterwards as this is much less likely to become dislodged. A surgeon must be present to perform a tracheostomy if intubation is not possible.

While the child is under the anaesthetic a blood culture and blood count can be done. Intravenous antibiotics should be started—chloramphenicol $(100 \, \text{mg} \, \text{kg}^{-1} \, (24 \, \text{h})^{-1})$ should be given in view of the

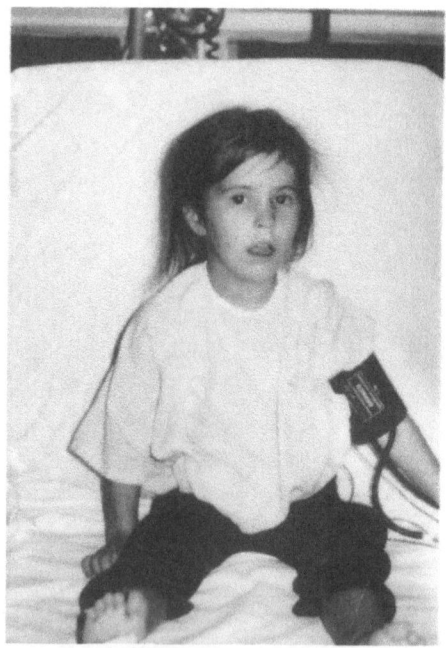

Figure 6 *At presentation—a six-year-old girl with epiglottitis who had a sore throat, high temperature and increasing respiratory distress for 8 hours*

possibility of ampicillin-resistant *Haemophilus influenzae*. As epi-glottitis is a life-threatening disorder chloramphenicol should be used initially and ampicillin $(400\,\text{mg}\,\text{kg}^{-1}\,(24\,\text{h})^{-1})$ can be given in addition, if desired. The chloramphenicol can be replaced by ampicillin once the sensitivity of the organism is known. The nasotracheal tube can usually be removed after 24 to 48 hours as recovery is usually very rapid once suitable antibiotics have been started. With careful and intensive treatment initiated early in the course of the illness a complete and rapid recovery can be expected. The course of the illness in a six-year-old girl is shown in Figures 6–8.

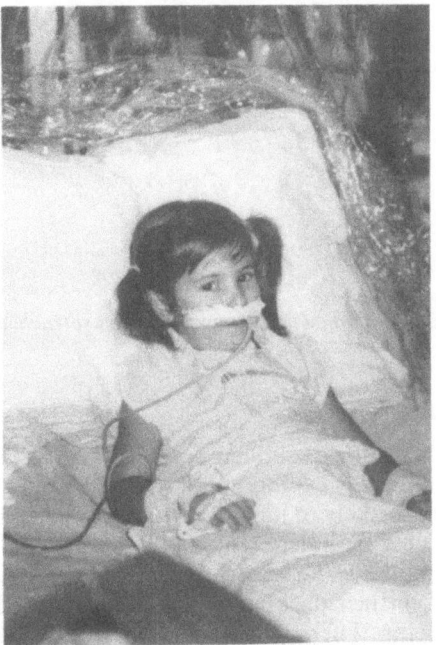

Figure 7 *At 24 hours, with a nasotracheal and nasogastric tube and an intravenous infusion* in situ

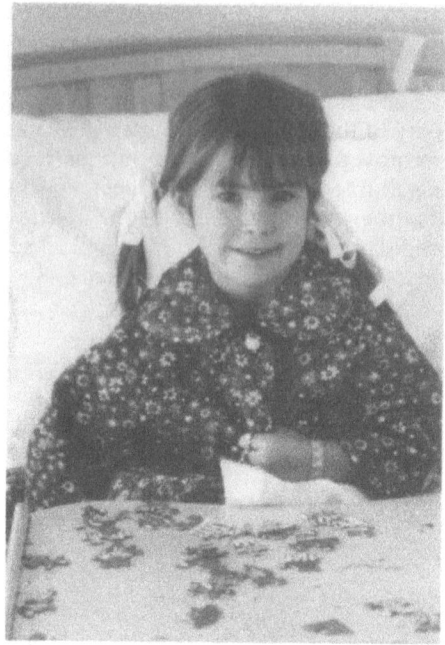

Figure 8   *At 72 hours following removal of the nasotracheal tube*

Foreign bodies

Any child with stridor of sudden onset may have inhaled a foreign body. Infants naturally explore small objects by putting them in their mouths—they are likely to inhale coins, safety-pins, beads and other household articles. Toddlers tend to inhale peanuts, fishbones and other foods (Figure 9). Peanuts are particularly troublesome as the organic oils from their decomposition cause marked bronchial irritation and oedema. There may be a history of choking or a sudden attack of coughing and any history suggesting that a foreign body may have been inhaled must never be ignored. However, the event may have taken place unobserved, so the absence of a definite history does not preclude the diagnosis.

The symptoms will depend on the size of the object inhaled and its location. Larger objects will impact proximally and cause obvious

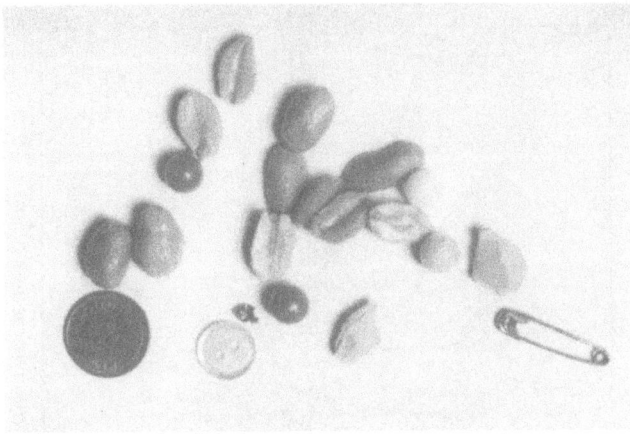

Figure 9 *Some foreign bodies commonly inhaled by infants and toddlers. Peanuts are the most common*

respiratory embarrassment immediately, whereas smaller particles lodging distally cause less dramatic symptoms and may not be detected for some time.

Severe upper airway obstruction

If there is severe airway obstruction caused by blockage in the larynx or trachea, the object needs to be removed urgently. It has recently been recommended that the child should be placed face downwards and given four blows to the back. This can be done most conveniently by placing the child across one's knees, or an infant over one's forearm. If this fails one should proceed to rapidly compress the chest four times, as if performing external cardiac massage. (American Academy of Pediatrics, First Aid for the Choking Child, 1981.) The Heimlich manœuvre, in which sudden compression of the upper abdomen forces the diaphragm upwards and propels the object out of the airway can also be used (Heimlich, 1975). It is most easily performed from behind the patient by placing one's hand on the upper abdomen and rapidly squeezing it. It is not though recommended by the American Academy of Pediatrics as damage to the viscera is more likely in children. If these procedures fail it may be possible to remove the object with a laryngoscope and forceps. If this

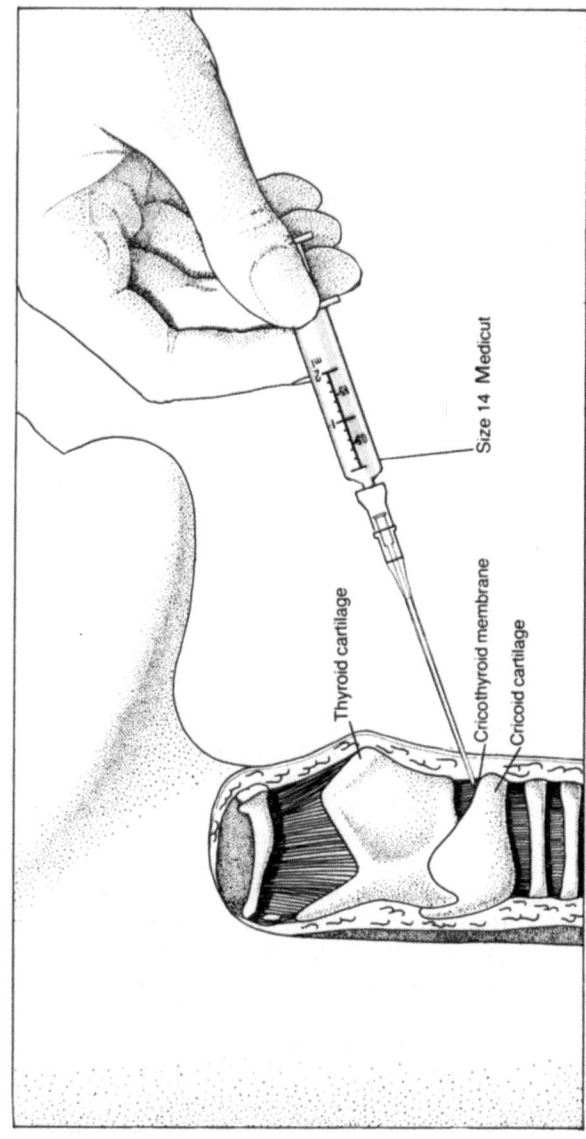

Figure 10 Site of insertion of the Medicut to relieve acute upper airways obstruction

is difficult and there is a risk of damaging the larynx or making the situation worse, it is better to establish an emergency airway. This can be done by inserting a wide-bore cannula, e.g. Medicut (size 12 or 14 French gauge) or with a pneumothorax trocar (size 12 French gauge) through the cricothyroid membrane (Figure 10). This will provide an airway until the object can be removed under anaesthesia.

Lower airways obstruction

The usual presentation is less acute, with a foreign body lodged in the bronchi or smaller airways. This may give rise to stridor or wheezing. The stridor tends to be softer than that of tracheal origin and has both an inspiratory and expiratory component. Examination may show asymmetrical chest movement with mediastinal shift, an area of decreased air entry or signs of pneumonia. A chest radiograph will show radio-opaque foreign bodies, but peanuts and other organic materials are radio-lucent. The commonest site of obstruction is the right main bronchus. There is often partial obstruction, acting like a ball-valve, which allows air entry on inspiration but not

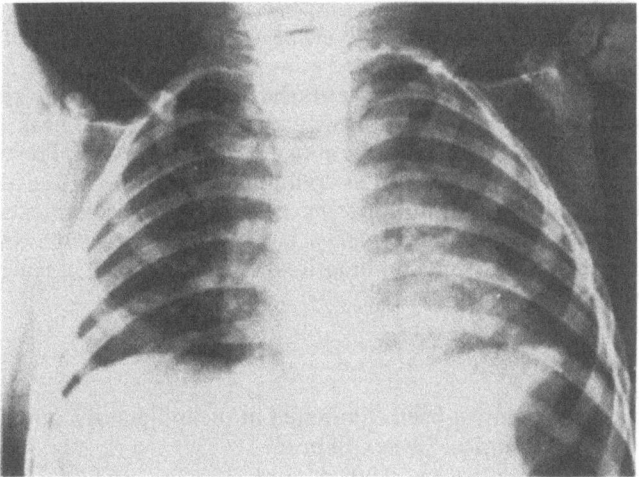

Figure 11   *This 3-year-old girl suddenly developed mild stridor 2 months before coming to hospital. She insisted on having her food cut into small pieces, but this was attributed to cussedness. The coin is lodged in the oesophagus*

on expiration, resulting in over-distension distally. For this to be appreciated radiographically, both inspiratory and expiratory films are needed as the expiratory film will highlight the over-inflated area of lung. These radiographs are often difficult to obtain in young children, and screening is more informative.

If the child can breathe it is best not to disturb him but to refer him for bronchoscopy. Slapping on the back or any other manœuvres may dislodge the object and result in more serious obstruction.

Even if the foreign body seems to have been ejected, follow-up radiographs and observation in hospital are usually advisable. Fragments may have been retained, or oedema may develop around the traumatized site. Foreign bodies which become lodged in the oesophagus may also impinge on the airway and cause stridor (Figure 11).

Retropharyngeal abscess

This once-common emergency is now very rare. It occurs in infants and young children when there is inflammation of the retropharyngeal lymph nodes following an upper respiratory tract infection. The infant has a high temperature and because of severe dysphagia refuses all feeds and has difficulty swallowing his saliva. He will hold his neck and head hyper-extended so as to achieve the optimal airway and frequently tilts his head towards the unaffected side. Any attempt to move the head will be vigorously opposed. A lateral neck radiograph will show swelling of the retropharyngeal space. Treatment, by surgical incision, is urgent as spontaneous rupture of the abscess is to be avoided and antibiotics need to be given. The most likely causative organisms are *Streptococci*, *Staphylococcus aureus* or anaerobic mouth flora, so a combination of penicillin and cloxacillin is suitable.

Diphtheria

Diphtheria has almost been eliminated in the indigenous population in Britain, but sporadic cases still occur.

It has a gradual onset, with a mild sore throat and moderate temperature. A greyish membrane forms on the tonsils which may extend to affect the larynx. This results in a cough, stridor and increasing dyspnoea. By this time the child will be severely ill, and death from laryngeal obstruction may follow unless a tracheostomy is performed and antitoxin and penicillin given.

Congenital laryngeal stridor

This is by far the most common cause of chronic stridor. In these children the epiglottis is long and the aryepiglottic folds long and floppy. During inspiration they collapse and cover the glottic area, causing obstruction and thereby producing stridor. The stridor usually begins shortly after birth, becoming more pronounced during the first few months of life. It gradually improves after a year and resolves by 18 months to 2 years. It is inspiratory, all but disappears with quiet breathing, but is aggravated by crying or excitement. The cry and cough are normal and there is no dysphagia. These children thrive perfectly well, but may suffer increased stridor when they have a URTI, when they should be treated as for laryngotracheobronchitis. If the child has stridor when at rest, or the voice is abnormal or there is dysphagia, direct laryngoscopy is indicated to identify vocal cord paralysis or lesions within the trachea, and a barium swallow to identify compression of the trachea from a vascular ring or a mediastinal mass.

Conclusion

Acute stridor is a sign which should never be ignored. An accurate diagnosis always needs to be made, so that appropriate treatment can be promptly initiated.

References

American Academy of Pediatrics (1981), First aid for the choking child, *Pediatrics*, **67**, 744.
Heimlich, H. J. (1975), *J. Am. Med. Assoc.*, **234**, 398.

Further reading

Barker, G. A. (1979), Controversies in the management of supraglottitis and croup. *Pediatric Clinics of North America*, **26**, 565.
Morus Jones, H. and Camps, F. (1957), Acute epiglottitis. *The Practitioner*, **178**, 223.
Williams, H. E. and Phelan, P. D. (1975), *Respiratory Illness in Children*, Blackwell Scientific Publications, Oxford.

CHAPTER 4

Lower respiratory tract disorders

Acute respiratory infections are the commonest illnesses in childhood and comprise almost half of all illnesses in children under 5 years (Figure 1). The preschool child has six to eight respiratory infections per year. Most of these are mild and in only two or three is there any constitutional upset. Most lower respiratory tract infections in children are viral and follow from infection of the upper respiratory tract. It is in the first year of life that lower respiratory tract infections are commonest and have the highest morbidity and mortality.

Infants

Epidemiological studies suggest that there is an increased incidence of lower respiratory tract infections in infants whose socioeconomic background is poor, if they live in an urban rather than a rural environment, if there is a sibling of preschool age, if their parents have respiratory symptoms, and if their mothers smoke (Figure 2) (Colley, 1976). Host factors of importance include congenital heart disease, congenital abnormalities of the lung, cystic fibrosis or immune deficiency.

An infant with a significant lower respiratory tract infection will frequently be reluctant to feed. Some constitutional disturbance will be present, as will signs of respiratory distress, such as flaring of the alae nasae, an abnormal pattern of respiration, tachypnoea and possibly cyanosis. Any serious lower respiratory tract infection in an

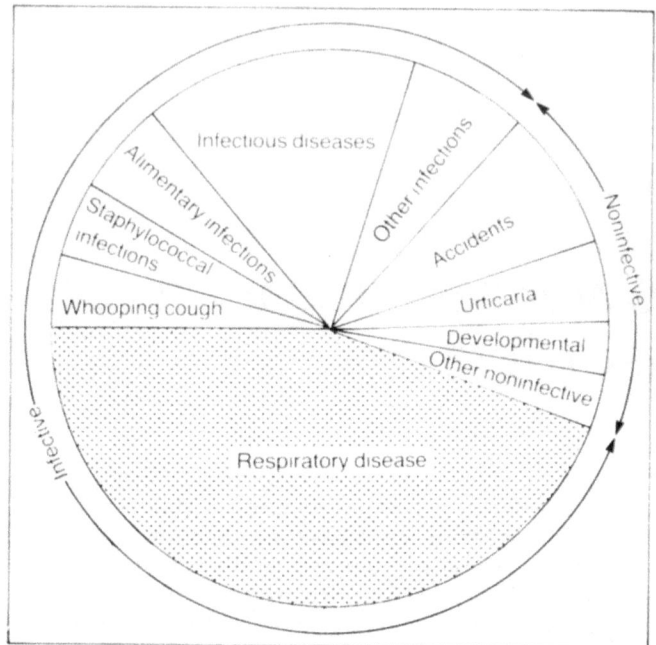

Figure 1   *The variety of illness in children during the first five years of life in Newcastle-upon-Tyne 1947–1952 (after Miller et al., 1960)*

infant will invariably be accompanied by tachypnoea at rest, when the respiratory rate is above 40/min, and this is a particularly useful sign. Supraclavicular, intercostal and substernal recession are pronounced when there is airways obstruction, as in bronchiolitis, but not in pneumonia when respiration tends to be shallow. Added sounds from secretions in the upper airways may be so widely conducted in the chest that they are not only easily audible but may also be felt. A chest radiograph must be taken whenever a significant lower respiratory infection is suspected, as there are often no localizing physical signs even in the presence of widespread consolidation.

Hypoxaemia occurs early in infants with lower respiratory tract infections There is a general reluctance to give children oxygen, perhaps because of the emphasis laid on the potential danger of giving it to elderly patients with chronic bronchitis who may rely on hypoxia for their respiratory drive. There is hardly ever this danger

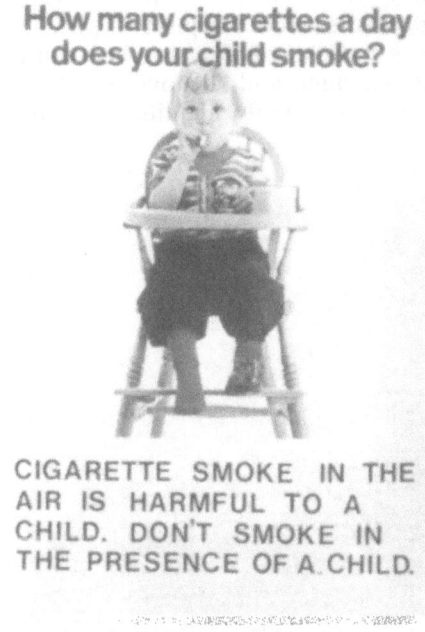

How many cigarettes a day does your child smoke?

CIGARETTE SMOKE IN THE AIR IS HARMFUL TO A CHILD. DON'T SMOKE IN THE PRESENCE OF A CHILD.

Figure 2 *There is an increased incidence of lower respiratory tract infections in infants whose mothers smoke (Fergusson et al., 1980)*

in giving oxygen to infants, and it may be life-saving. In the seriously ill infant, respiratory function is more accurately assessed by blood gas analysis. Unfortunately, in spite of using local anaesthesia, infants often cry during the procedure, and this will reduce the arterial oxygen tension and make interpretation of the results more difficult. When serial measurements are needed, an arterial line (usually in the radial or dorsalis pedis arteries) allows intermittent sampling without disturbing the child.

As in any seriously ill infant, the disease may not be confined to the chest and other sites of infection should be sought.

Bronchiolitis

Bronchiolitis is the commonest serious lower respiratory infection of infants, and mainly affects infants less than a year old, with a peak incidence between two and six months. It occurs in epidemics between December and April. Respiratory syncytial virus (RSV) is responsible in over 70% of cases—other causes include para-influenza, influenza, rhino and adenoviruses. RSV in nasopharyngeal secretions can be rapidly identified by immunofluorescence (Figure 3).

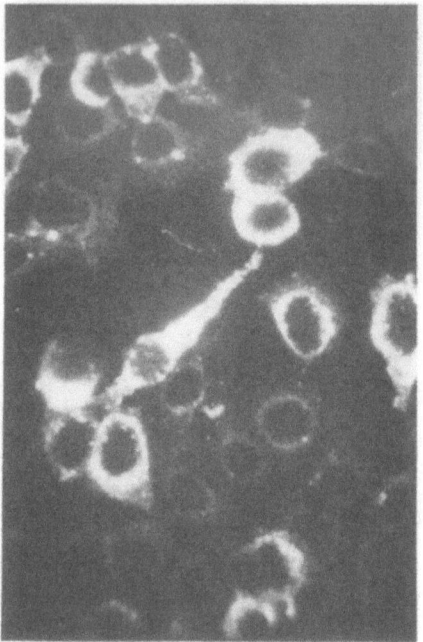

Figure 3 *Respiratory syncytial virus from a nasopharyngeal aspirate demonstrated by indirect immunofluorescence*

Pathophysiology

Inflammation of the bronchioles occurs with oedema, loss of cilia, necrosis of the epithelial cells and obstruction of the lumen by cellular debris and thick secretions. This bronchiolar obstruction is patchy and results in some areas of overinflation and others of atelectasis, causing marked ventilation–perfusion mismatch.

Clinical features

Typically the illness starts with coryzal symptoms, and over the next two to three days a characteristic, irritating cough, tachypnoea and difficulty in feeding develop. The infant is usually afebrile and not toxic. If the disease progresses there is increasing tachypnoea with use of the accessory muscles of respiration. The chest becomes barrel-shaped because of hyperinflation, and the liver is displaced downwards. There are widespread fine inspiratory crepitations over the entire lung fields which may be accompanied by expiratory wheezes. The typical findings on the chest radiograph are of hyper-lucent lung fields and flattening of the diaphragms. There may also be some perihilar bronchial thickening typical of viral infections and patchy areas of collapse. Apnoeic attacks may occur, and, if they are the presenting feature, may resemble near-miss sudden infant death syndrome.

Management

Management is supportive and directed at assessing the respiratory status and preventing respiratory failure. The respiratory rate is the best clinical guide to hypoxaemia and the course of the illness. At a respiratory rate of 60/min, the Pao_2 will have dropped to about 8 kPa (60 mmHg) and will drop even further with a higher respiratory rate (Reynolds, 1963). Hypoxia is usually relieved by giving 30 to 40% oxygen. Humidified oxygen can be given by placing the baby in a chair in a transparent oxygen tent, or in a chair with a head box or, in the very young, in an incubator. The oxygen concentration within the tent should be monitored to ensure that an adequate level is maintained, as leaks are common. There is no advantage in adding mist into the tent, as the lower airways are fully saturated and the condensation makes observation more difficult.

Careful observation and monitoring are required. Cyanosis in air, increasing respiratory distress (a respiratory rate above 60/min and rising), and diminished breath sounds are signs of severe disease and indicate the need for blood gas estimation. Artificial ventilation of these infants requires considerable skill and is hazardous. The indications for its use are mainly clinical. Most infants with a $Paco_2$ greater than 8.5 kPa (65 mmHg) will require intermittent positive pressure ventilation, as will any infant with a reduced level of consciousness. Immediate intubation may also be required for apnoeic attacks.

Hydration

Most infants cannot maintain an adequate fluid intake by mouth because of their respiratory distress. In milder cases and during recovery small quantities of milk can be given frequently by naso-gastric tube, but this has the disadvantages of obstructing one nostril which increases the work of breathing, and any vomiting may result in aspiration. Alternatively an orogastric tube can be used, but they are more easily dislodged. In severe cases intravenous hydration will be required. Overhydration should be avoided, as inappropriate ADH production is not uncommon and the negative intrathoracic pressures generated during maximum respiratory efforts may predispose to pulmonary oedema. Initially it is wisest to give the normal maintenance fluid requirements only, unless the baby is dehydrated.

Drugs

Antibiotics are not indicated as bronchiolitis is a viral disease, although they may be given if there is difficulty in differentiating it from bacterial bronchopneumonia, particularly if the infant is very ill. Double-blind studies have failed to reveal any benefit from steroids.

Cardiac failure

Cardiac failure tends to be overdiagnosed in infants with bronchiolitis as in both conditions there is tachypnoea, tachycardia and the liver is palpable several centimetres below the right costal margin. Cardiac failure rarely occurs in infants with bronchiolitis unless they have congenital heart disease, and is indicated by excessive weight gain, a gallop rhythm, an enlarging heart and pulmonary oedema on chest radiographs.

Prognosis

Most infants recover in seven to ten days. The relationship between bronchiolitis and asthma and atopy is controversial. Minor abnormalities in respiratory function can still be detected many years after an attack of bronchiolitis, and there is an increased incidence of coughing and wheezing. It appears that only a small proportion of affected children develop asthma.

Pneumonia

Viruses are responsible for most cases of pneumonia in childhood (Table 1). Bacterial infections also produce serious disease, usually caused by the pneumococcus and, rarely, by *Staphylococcus aureus*, *Haemophilus influenzae* and Group A β-haemolytic streptococci. Gram-negative bacilli including *Escherichia coli* and *Pseudomonas* are also found in infants less than two months old, those with impaired immunity or those requiring artificial ventilation (Table 2).

Table 1   Viral causes of pneumonia in young children

Viral	
Respiratory syncytial virus ⎫	
Para-influenza ⎬	Common
Influenza ⎭	
Adenovirus ⎫	
Rhinovirus ⎭	Infrequent

Table 2   Important causes of pneumonia in children at different ages

<2 months	*2 months–5 years*	*>5 years*
Gram-negative organisms	Viral (see Table 1)	Viral
Group B β-haemolytic streptococcus	Pneumococcal *H. influenzae*	Pneumococcal *Mycoplasma pneumoniae*
Staphylococcus aureus	Group A β-haemolytic streptococci *Staphylococcus aureus*	

Viral pneumonias

Respiratory syncytial virus, para-influenza, influenza and adenovirus may spread down the respiratory tract. The clinical picture ranges from the common mild illness to the fulminant. In young children there are often few abnormal signs on auscultation, with perhaps only a few scattered crepitations, but patchy consolidation is seen on the chest radiograph.

Mycoplasma pneumoniae

This predominantly affects the older child aged between five and fifteen years. General malaise, headache, fever, cough and mucoid sputum are characteristic. On auscultation fine crepitations may be heard, but the chest signs tend to be unimpressive compared to the degree of lassitude. Changes on the chest radiograph are variable— there may be widespread diffuse shadowing, or lobar or segmental consolidation. The diagnosis can be confirmed by culturing the organism or from serum antibodies. The disease may follow a protracted course.

Pneumococcal pneumonia

The symptoms and signs at presentation may not be very specific, with a toxic child with high fever and delirium. Rapid, grunting respirations may suggest chest disease but localizing signs of dullness to percussion, crepitations and bronchial breathing may be entirely absent or difficult to detect, and a chest radiograph is needed to make the diagnosis. Whereas the chest radiograph may show consolidation of lobar distribution in the older child (Figure 4), it is often patchy in the infant. The organism may be identified on blood culture. Headache and neck stiffness accompanying upper lobe consolidation may make one suspect meningitis, and abdominal pain from consolidation of the lower lobes can be sufficiently severe to mimic an acute abdominal emergency.

Staphylococcal pneumonia

Staphylococcal pneumonia is now rarely seen but is important in view of its severity and the high incidence of complications. Infants

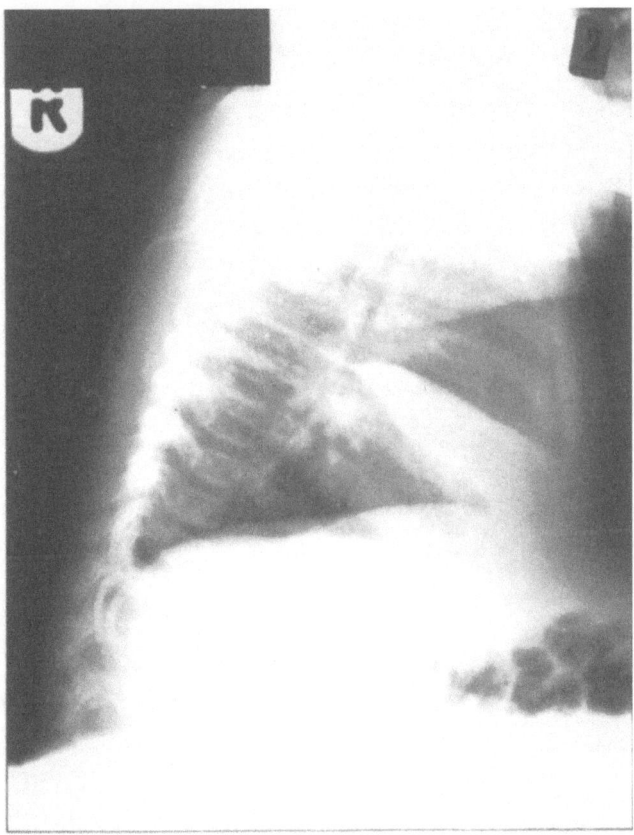

Figure 4 *A lateral chest radiograph showing right middle lobe collapse and consolidation, suggesting pneumococcal pneumonia*

and debilitated children are particularly vulnerable. It tends to be acute, causing severe toxicity which may proceed to shock. On auscultation, many will have widespread coarse crepitations, and there may be signs of hyperinflation. The chest radiograph may show scattered areas of consolidation throughout both lung fields, or more commonly, a large dense area with one or more pneumatocoeles, which are thin-walled cavities containing air (Figure 5). Pleural

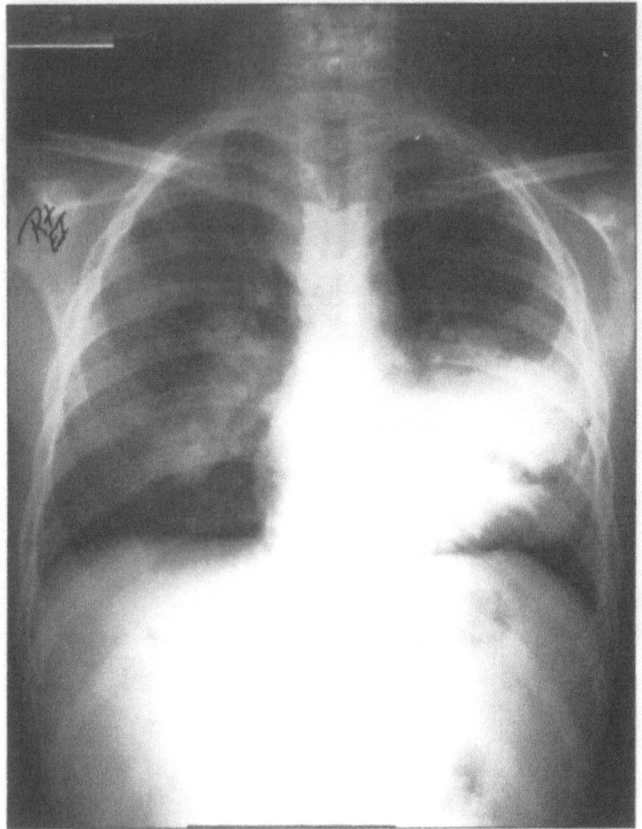

Figure 5 *A chest radiograph in staphylococcal pneumonia showing extensive consolidation and a pneumatocoele*

effusions and empyema may be present. Other complications include tension pneumothorax and respiratory failure.

Management of pneumonia

Most infants and young children with pneumonia require admission to hospital, while many older children can be managed at home. This depends on the degree of constitutional disturbance, respiratory distress and home circumstances.

Careful monitoring and supportive measures as described for bronchiolitis are required. Although viruses are the major causes of pneumonia in infants and young children they cannot be readily distinguished from bacterial pneumonia and treatment with antibiotics should be given.

In most cases the choice of antibiotic will be determined by the clinical features, particularly the severity of the illness, the child's age and the appearance of the chest radiograph. Investigations to identify the organism responsible are seldom of help in deciding on the initial treatment. Sputum is rarely obtained in children. Throat swabs are seldom of assistance in identifying bacterial pathogens as asymptomatic children are often carriers of the pneumococcus and *Haemophilus influenzae*. Neutrophilia and a 'left shift' are suggestive of a bacterial infection but are non-specific. Blood cultures may be positive if the child is septicaemic but this information is only available 24–48 hours later. Respiratory syncytial virus can be identified rapidly by immunofluorescence if this service is available, but the results of viral cultures or viral antibodies are only available after a long delay.

In infants less than two months old Gram-negative organisms and Group B β-haemolytic streptococci and rarely *Staphylococcus aureus* may be responsible. Ampicillin or cloxacillin (Orbenin) together with gentamicin (Genticin) should be given parenterally.

In children under two years old, the pneumococcus is probably the most common bacterial pathogen, but *Staphylococcus aureus* and *Haemophilus influenzae* must be considered. Ampicillin (Penbritin) or amoxycillin (Amoxil) is often used, and cloxacillin (Orbenin) added if infection with *Staphylococcus aureus* is considered possible. If the infant is seriously ill, the same combination of antibiotics as described for very young infants should be given.

In children between two and five years old amoxycillin (Amoxil) or co-trimoxazole (Septrin, Bactrim) to include cover for *Haemophilus influenzae* are often used. If there is lobar consolidation suggesting pneumococcal pneumonia, penicillin is the drug of choice and may need to be given intravenously*. When the clinical features are

---

* Whenever children with pneumonia are seriously ill the antibiotics should be given parenterally.

suggestive of *Mycoplasma pneumoniae*, erythromycin (Erythrocin) is the antibiotic of choice.

Delay in resolution may be associated with the presence of foreign bodies, underlying congenital abnormalities, cystic fibrosis (Figure 6) or immune deficiency. Tuberculosis (Figure 7) must always be considered, and all children with pneumonia should have a tuberculin skin test. Unusual organisms may be the cause of pneumonia, for example, *Pneumocystis carinii* or cytomegalovirus in immunosuppressed children, and *Chlamydia trachomatis* has been described as a rare cause of pneumonia in infants.

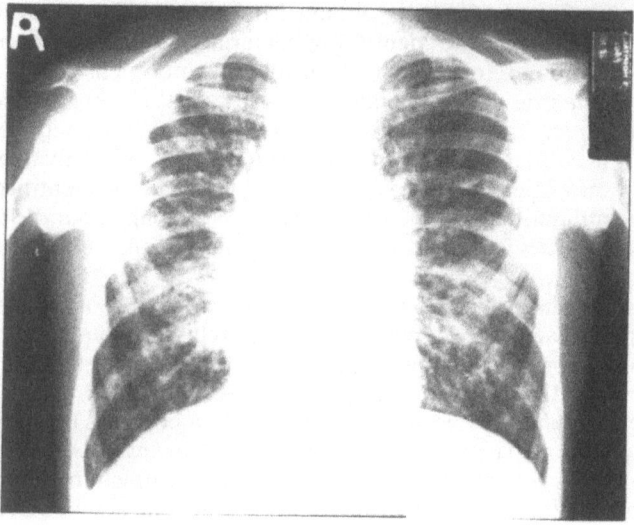

Figure 6 *Chest radiograph of an eight-year-old boy with cystic fibrosis, who initially presented with pneumonia as an infant. He has extensive changes, including bronchial line shadowing and many ring shadows from abscess cavities*

Pertussis

The number of children who receive pertussis immunization has dropped dramatically following the adverse publicity that pertussis immunization may be associated with neurological damage. Since then there has been an increased incidence of clinical cases, and

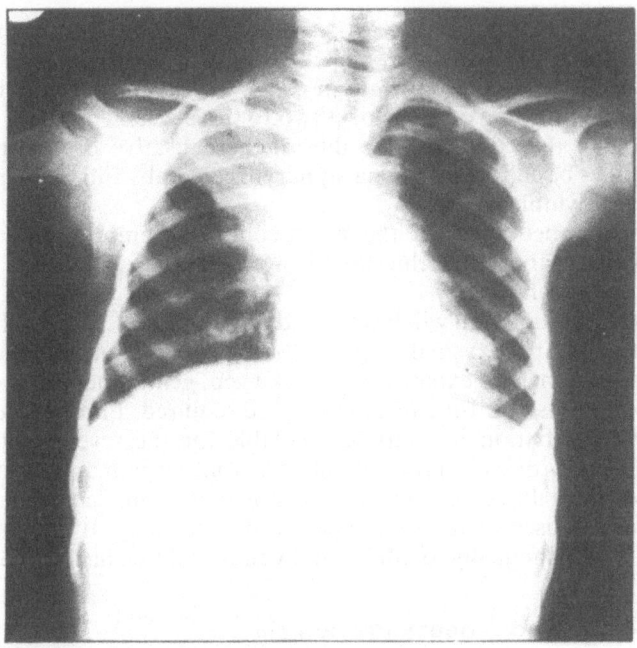

Figure 7 *Chest radiograph of a child with tuberculosis showing consolidation and hilar lymphadenopathy*

during 1978 there was a severe epidemic with 66 000 cases and 11 deaths notified. Pertussis is particularly dangerous in infants less than six months old, and has a high mortality rate in countries where malnutrition is common. The clinical course follows a set sequence. The catarrhal stage lasts for one to two weeks during which the disease is most infectious. The dry cough becomes increasingly severe and paroxysmal. Spasms of coughing may be followed by an inspiratory 'whoop' in older children, but this is often absent in infants. Paroxysms are more marked at night, and may be provoked by crying, feeding or any disturbance. At the end of the paroxysm, vomiting may occur, and the child may develop facial congestion or become cyanosed or apnoeic. These apnoeic spells may also occur independently of the spasms of coughing and this is a particular problem in young babies. Severe conjunctival haemorrhages and facial petechiae due to raised venous pressure are dramatic features

67

but resolve spontaneously. More serious are convulsions from asphyxia, and rarely, intracranial bleeding or encephalopathy. This 'spasmodic' phase lasts from four to six weeks, and the cough then gradually improves over the next two to three weeks.

Early in the course of the illness, the causative organism may sometimes be cultured from nasopharyngeal swabs and there may be a marked lymphocytosis.

Bronchopneumonia is the most common complication, particularly in infants. Bronchiectasis is a well recognized sequel, but is now rarely seen.

Hospital admission will be required for the more seriously affected infant at the paroxysmal stage of the illness. The most important part of treatment is expert nursing. Oxygen, gentle suction of excessive secretions and tube feeding may be required. Facilities for immediate intubation need to be available for the severely affected infant. Erythromycin given at the catarrhal stage may modify the course of the illness, but the diagnosis is seldom made at this stage. It is mainly used to reduce the period of infectivity. It may also be given prophylactically to infants and young children in close contact.

Wheezing and wheezy bronchitis

Viral upper respiratory tract infections often spread to involve the bronchial mucosa. Cough is usually the only symptom of lower tract involvement and constitutional upset is only slight. The respiratory rate is normal or only marginally increased, and the only abnormal signs on auscultation are a few coarse crepitations from increased secretions and sometimes mild wheezing. These children are usually

Table 3   Some important causes of wheezing in infants and children

Asthma/wheezy bronchitis
Bronchiolitis
Laryngotracheobronchitis
Aspiration of milk or food
Cystic fibrosis
Inhaled foreign body
Extrinsic congestion e.g. lymph nodes (TB), tumour, foreign body in oesophagus
Congenital—vascular rings
          —tracheal webs and stenosis

said to have 'bronchitis' but if the wheezing is pronounced in young children it is often referred to as 'wheezy bronchitis'. It is difficult to predict which children with wheezy bronchitis will go on to develop asthma, but most do not. The family history and other manifestations of atopy are not different in children with wheezy bronchitis who do not develop asthma from children with asthma. However, the older a child is at the onset of wheezing, the more likely he is to develop asthma.

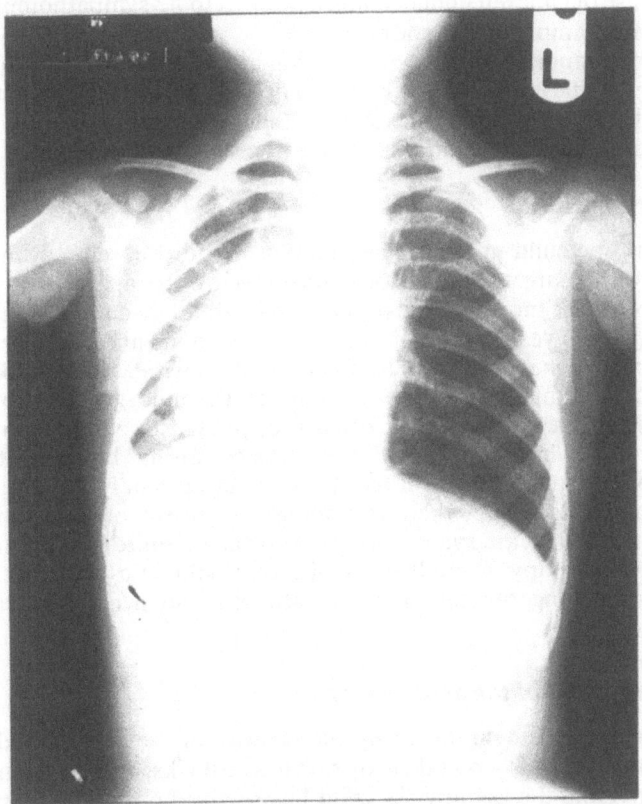

Figure 8 *Chest radiograph of a 16-month-old boy who was noted to be wheezing three days after choking on a peanut. There is air trapping on the left with a shift of the mediastinum. A peanut was removed from the left main bronchus*

Follow-up studies have shown that only 3-7% of children who were wheezing at under one year became asthmatic. Most had only one or two episodes of wheezy bronchitis. Of those who had their first attack between one and three years old, 18% became asthmatic, while 42% of those who had their first attack after the age of three years became asthmatic (Boesen, 1953). Antibiotics do not alter the course of wheezy bronchitis, and should not be prescribed. Bronchodilators, e.g. salbutamol (Ventolin) may be indicated, but the response of children under eighteen months to β_2-sympathomimetics like salbutamol may be poor.

Other important causes of wheezing are listed in Table 3. Inhaled foreign bodies, especially peanuts, may result in wheezing (Figure 8). It is being increasingly recognized that recurrent aspiration from gastro-oesophageal reflux can cause wheezing in infants.

Acute asthma

About one child in twenty has asthma. A third develop symptoms before they are two years old and most by the age of five years. Although the mortality is extremely low, about 40 children die from asthma each year in the UK, with the very young and adolescents at particular risk. It is helpful to divide children with asthma into three groups. About three-quarters belong to the mild group who have acute episodes of wheezing, often precipitated by viral respiratory infections, whose lung function returns to normal between attacks and who require treatment for the acute attacks only. In a quarter, the moderate group, there is some derangement of lung function even when they are symptom-free, and they require long-term prophylactic therapy. A small group of severe asthmatics have markedly abnormal lung function between attacks, and need maintenance steroids.

Management of the acute attack

Management is determined by the severity of the acute attack but account must also be taken of previous attacks, their response to therapy, and the therapy the child has received both long-term and in the previous few hours. Arrival in hospital often provides reassurance for both the child and parents and may be accompanied by improvement. Parents should be encouraged to seek help early in an attack, and an efficient system is required to ensure that the child is seen promptly and treatment instituted. The child should be disturbed as little as possible apart from essential observations and investigations.

Clinical features

A hacking cough, dyspnoea with prolonged expiration and a high pitched wheeze are early features. Breathing against increasing airways obstruction will be manifest by the increasing use of the accessory muscles of respiration, with supraclavicular, intercostal and substernal retractions and hyperexpansion of the chest. As the attack becomes more severe, the child's breathlessness makes speaking difficult and the wheezing becomes both expiratory and inspiratory. Ominous signs are cyanosis in spite of receiving oxygen, if the respiratory rate and pulse continue to rise, if there is reduced air entry or a decrease in the wheeze which is not accompanied by clinical improvement and a deterioration in the level of consciousness.

Initial therapy

A flow diagram is shown in Figure 9 and the drugs used listed in Table 4. Initial therapy is with a selective β_2-sympathomimetic agent

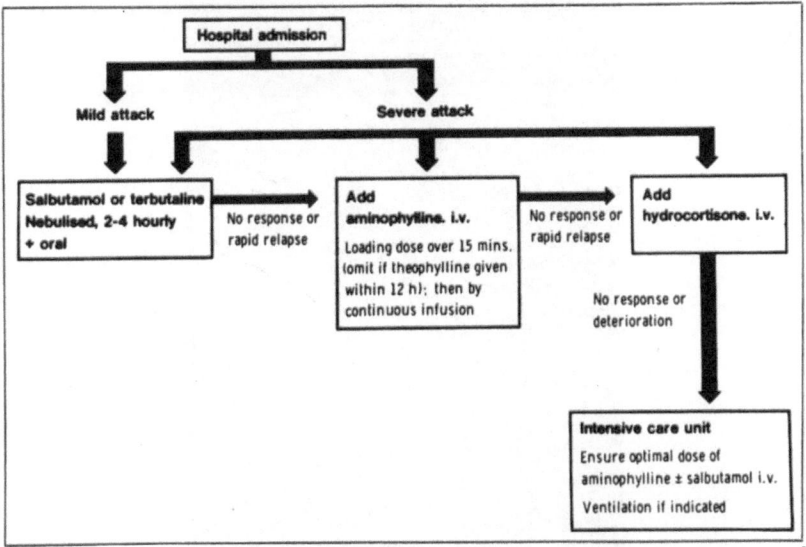

Figure 9 *Flow diagram for the management of severe asthma in hospital*

Table 4 Drugs in acute asthma

Drug	Route	Frequency	Dose
Salbutamol	Nebulizer	2–4-hourly	0.5 to 1.5 ml of 0.5% ventilator solution made up to 2 ml with normal saline
	i.v.	Hourly	5 to 7×10^{-3} mg/kg
Terbutaline	s.c.	6-hourly	0.005 mg/kg (0.01 ml/kg)
	Nebulizer	2–4-hourly	2 to 5 mg
Aminophylline	i.v.	Loading dose over 20 min	5 to 6 mg/kg
	i.v.	Continuous infusion	$1 \, \text{mg} \, \text{kg}^{-1} \text{h}^{-1}$ if <9 y $0.7 \, \text{mg} \, \text{kg}^{-1} \text{h}^{-1}$ if >9 y
Hydrocortisone	i.v.	2–4-hourly	100–200 mg
Prednisolone	p.o.	Daily	1–2 mg/kg initially. Tail off over five to seven days

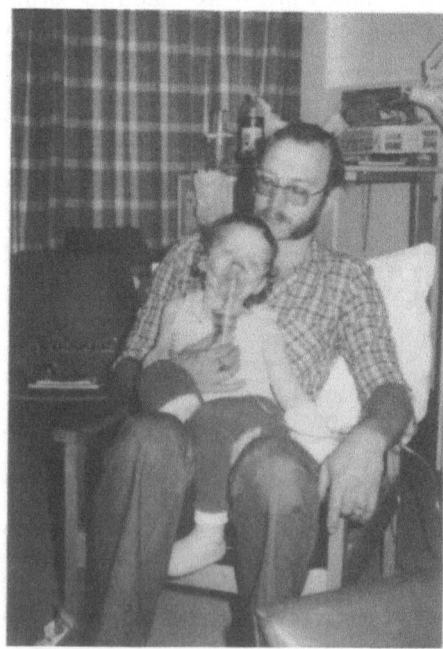

Figure 10 *A young child with asthma sitting on her father's knee receiving nebulized salbutamol via a face mask*

(salbutamol or terbutaline) given as a nebulized solution via either a face mask or a mouth piece. Young children may initially be frightened by the apparatus, but demonstration with their parent's help will usually persuade them to use it (Figure 10). This treatment has superseded subcutaneous adrenaline as the first-line therapy for an acute attack as it is safer and does not involve an injection. Many children will respond completely to one or two inhalations of the nebulizer and will be able to go home on oral therapy, while those with more severe attacks need to be admitted.

Hospital admission

Many children even in hospital can be managed with a β_2-sympathomimetic agent given regularly via a nebulizer and orally. Progress can be monitored by measuring the peak expiratory flow rate with a Wright's peak flow meter.

The response of children under 18 months to β_2-sympathomimetics is often disappointing, but an improvement is seen in some of them. Children who still have respiratory distress after the nebulized bronchodilator will require intravenous therapy.

Intravenous drug therapy

Aminophylline is given to those who do not respond to the nebulized salbutamol and is administered slowly over 15 to 20 minutes to avoid the dangers of nausea and vomiting, cardiac dysrhythmias and convulsions. Thereafter it can be given by constant infusion. All these children should be on a cardiac monitor. If an aminophylline-containing preparation has been used within the preceding 12 hours, the loading dose should be omitted or the serum aminophylline level measured first. Alternatively, intravenous salbutamol can be given. As absorption of aminophylline from rectal suppositories is erratic, they should not be used.

Steroids will be required if the child has not responded to nebulized salbutamol and intravenous aminophylline. Hydrocortisone should be given intravenously initially but takes a few hours to achieve its maximum effect. It should also be given if the child is already on oral steroids or has recently received a course of steroids. Oral prednisolone can be substituted when the acute attack is subsiding and is usually given as a short course in reducing doses over five to seven days.

The drugs have been described sequentially but in a severely ill child they should be given simultaneously and immediately.

Investigations

Children who still have respiratory distress after the initial therapy with the nebulizer and intravenous drugs should have a chest radiograph and arterial blood gases performed. Blood gases are probably done less often than they should be, as one is reluctant to disturb and upset children. Particularly in the young child, the true severity of the physiological disturbance as shown by blood gas estimation may easily be underestimated from clinical criteria (McKenzie et al., 1979). Hypoxia occurs early, but the Pa_{CO_2} is initially low because of hyperventilation. Only in severe cases is the Pa_{CO_2} raised, and at this stage there is also a metabolic acidosis secondary to hypoxia, poor peripheral perfusion and dehydration (Table 5). A chest radiograph will be required to detect a pneumothorax, pneumomediastinum or pneumonia. Although some of the children will be too dyspnoeic to be able to perform a peak expiratory flow rate on admission, it can be used subsequently to assess their progress provided they are old enough to use the flow meter (Figure 10).

Table 5   Assessing the severity of respiratory distress by arterial blood gases

Degree of obstruction	Pa_{O_2}	Pa_{CO_2}	Acid–base balance
+ +	↓	↓	Respiratory alkalosis
+ + +	↓ ↓	Normal	Normal
+ + + +	↓ ↓ ↓	↓	Respiratory plus metabolic acidosis

Supportive therapy

Oxygen is required for any child who is cyanosed. For children less than 18 months old this is best given in an oxygen tent and for those over five years old, by face mask. For children between these ages either method can be tried but they tend to be poorly tolerated.

Water loss from the respiratory tract is markedly increased and

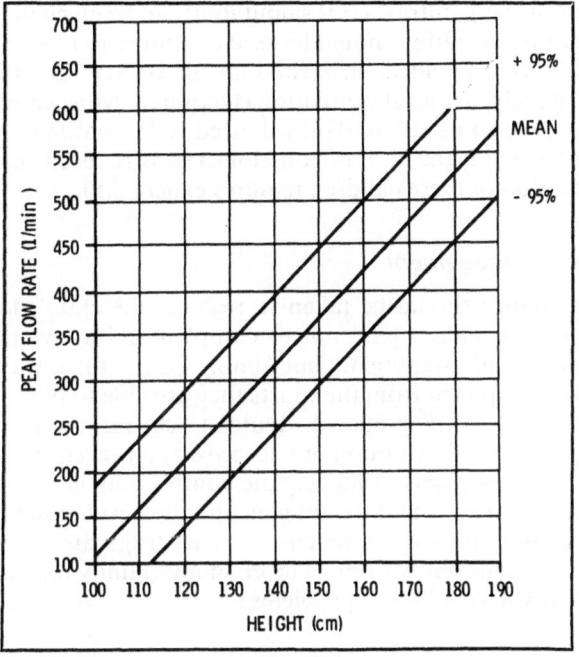

Figure 11 *Peak flow rate in normal children measured with a Wright peak flow meter. (Reproduced with permission from Godfrey, 1970)*

this is accompanied by poor fluid intake. As in bronchiolitis, there are dangers associated with overhydration, and usually only maintenance intravenous fluids (with 4% dextrose/0.18% saline) are advisable.

In contrast to adults it is rare for the attacks to be precipitated by bacterial infections, and antibiotics do not affect the outcome. They are indicated only if there is evidence of pneumonia.

Intensive care unit

Children who are severely ill on admission or who deteriorate after the initial therapy will need to be managed in an intensive care unit. The blood level of aminophylline should be monitored to ensure that it is in the high therapeutic range. Levels above this are associated with an increased incidence of side effects. If the child's condition is still not improving, intravenous salbutamol can be given in addition. Whether or not sedation should be used continues to be debated, but it is usually best avoided. Bronchial lavage is very seldom used in children. Rarely, artificial ventilation is required. Most children with a $Pa\text{CO}_2$ above 8 kPa (60 mmHg) will need to be ventilated, and it is always indicated if the level of consciousness is reduced. Intubation and ventilation of these children requires expert skill.

Long-term management

The opportunity should be taken to reassess the child's long-term management. Children tend not to complain about symptoms resulting from undertreatment, but simply adapt their way of life. Clues can be obtained from the sports they are able to play and from the amount of schooling missed. Acute attacks may be precipitated by infection, exercise, emotion or allergens, and preventive measures may be indicated. Signs of inadequate control may be suggested by unsatisfactory growth and weight gain and the development of chest deformity. It is important to ensure that drugs are being taken properly and sufficiently often. The child and family may also need help with any psychological problems.

References

Colley, J.R.T. (1976), in: *Recent Advances in Paediatrics, No. 5*, Hull, D. (Ed.), Churchill Livingstone, Edinburgh.

Fergusson, D.M., Horwood, L.J., Shannon, F.T. (1980), *Arch. Dis. Child.*, **55**, 358.

Godfrey, S. (1970), *Br. J. Dis. Chest*, **64**, 15.

Miller, F.J.W., Court, S.D.M., Walton, W.S. and Knox, E.G. (1960), *Growing up in Newcastle-upon-Tyne*, Oxford University Press, London.

McKenzie, S.A., Edmunds, A.T. and Godfrey, S. (1979), *Arch. Dis. Child.*, **54**, 581.

Reynolds, E.O.R. (1963), *Br. Med. J.*, **1**, 1192.

Further reading

Clark, T.J.H. and Godfrey, S. (1977), *Asthma*, Chapman and Hall, London.

Williams, H.E. and Phelan, P.D. (1975), *Respiratory Illness in Children*, Blackwell Scientific Publications, Oxford.

CHAPTER 5

Diarrhoea and vomiting

The consequences of diarrhoea and vomiting are much more serious in infants than they are in adults. Infants are particularly susceptible to dehydration because of their very high turnover of water relative to their size. An infant's normal fluid intake of 120 to 150 ml/kg each day represents 12 to 15% of his body weight. The fluid deficit sustained by a baby with only a moderate bout of gastroenteritis is considerable and equivalent to a severe attack of cholera in an adult. It is for this reason that infants with diarrhoea and vomiting need to be handled with great care.

The frequency and consistency of stools passed by normal infants varies widely, from firm stools every few days to loose motions every couple of hours. In particular, the stools of breast-fed infants may be loose, pale, occasionally green, and very frequent. Starvation stools may also be green and contain little faecal material. Gastroenteritis

Table 1   Common causes of acute diarrhoea

Infections	*Surgical conditions*
Gastroenteritis	Appendicitis
Urinary tract infection	Intussusception
Respiratory tract infection	
Meningitis	*Miscellaneous*
Septicaemia	Drugs, e.g. ampicillin
	Cows' milk protein intolerance
	Coeliac disease

is by far the commonest cause of diarrhoea of acute onset in infants, but other causes are listed in Table 1. Diarrhoea often occurs as a nonspecific feature of urinary and respiratory tract infections, otitis media and meningitis. It is also important to exclude a surgical condition, in particular intussusception and appendicitis.

Gastroenteritis

Gastroenteritis is a major cause of childhood death throughout the world. The malnourished infant is particularly vulnerable and in developing countries gastroenteritis causes millions of deaths every year. In Britain the incidence and mortality have decreased markedly but it remains among the five most common causes of hospital admission in children. It is rarely seen in infants who are totally breast-fed.

Aetiology

The relative importance of the different organisms responsible for gastroenteritis varies widely from country to country. Relatively recently, it has been established that viruses are the major pathogens in this country. Rotavirus is the commonest and was identified initially by electron microscopy of stools. Its name is derived from its resemblance to a wheel (Figure 1). Table 2 compares some of the clinical features of those diseases caused by the common organisms. In many cases no pathogen can be identified. Only a few important features will be discussed in more detail.

Rotavirus. Gastroenteritis caused by rotavirus mainly affects infants betweeen six months and two years old and is particularly prevalent during the winter. In two-thirds of cases, gastrointestinal symptoms are preceded by respiratory symptoms, usually with an upper respiratory tract infection with a cough and nasal discharge; there may be fever and otitis media. This is almost always followed by vomiting and then diarrhoea, which is watery and free of blood. The vomiting lasts between one and three days, while the diarrhoea lasts for about five days. The vomiting usually settles with clear fluids but the diarrhoea lasts several days irrespective of the method of rehydration (Lewis *et. al.,* 1979). The virus reduces the disaccharidase activity and there may be blunting of the villi of the small intestine, and virus

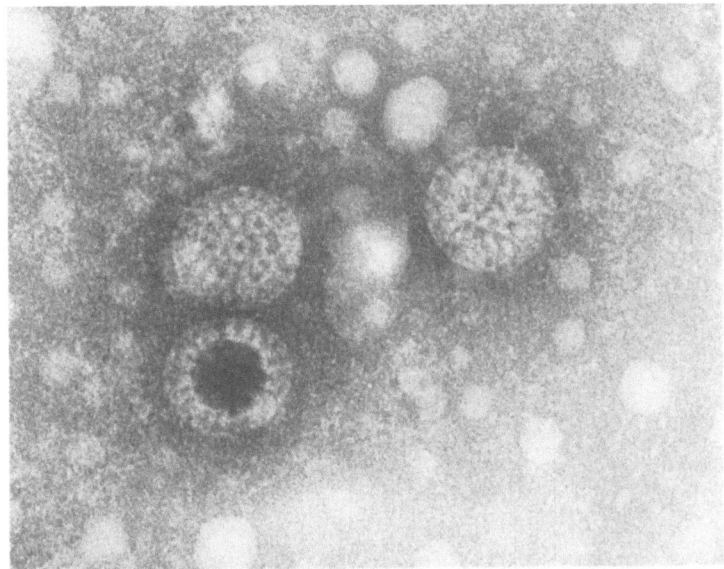

Figure 1 *Electron micrograph showing rotaviruses in stools. Rotavirus is the commonest identified cause of gastroenteritis in infants*

particles can be found within the villous cytoplasm: it may be that the five-day duration of the diarrhoea represents the generation time of a new villous epithelium (*British Medical Journal*, 1980). The most severe symptoms are found in infants, although rotavirus can be found in all age groups; symptoms tend to be mild in the neonatal period. It is highly infectious and may spread rapidly.

Shigella is notable for causing a high fever which may be accompanied by a convulsion. The diarrhoea may be profuse and contains blood and polymorphs.

Campylobacter. Following the introduction of selective culture techniques, *Campylobacter* has been recognized as an important cause of gastroenteritis in infants and children. The clinical features are variable, ranging from insignificant diarrhoea to severe diarrhoea often containing blood. A particular feature is abdominal pain which may resemble an acute abdomen.

Table 2 Typical clinical features of the common causes of gastroenteritis (Adapted from Barnes and Roberton 1979)

	Shigella	Escherichia coli	Salmonella	Campylobacter	Rotavirus
Age	6 m to 5 years	Under 2 years	Any	Any	Under 2 years
Diarrhoea in household	50%	No	Variable	Variable (including pets)	Variable
Incubation	24 to 72 hours	24 to 48 hours	8 to 24 hours	2 to 5 days	48 to 72 hours
Vomiting	Absent	±	Common	±	Common
High fever	Common	Absent	±	±	Common
Respiratory symptoms	25%	Absent	Absent	Absent	URTI in 65%
Fits	10%	Absent	Rare	Absent	Uncommon
Pain	Common	Rare	Variable	Marked	Rare
Stools					
Blood	+++	−	++	++	−
Mucus	++	±	++	±	−
Polymorphs	+++	−	++	−	−

Clinical assessment

The main dangers of gastroenteritis are dehydration and electrolyte imbalance which may cause death. For this reason it is important to ascertain the severity of the illness and the child's level of hydration. The degree of dehydration is usually described in terms of mass of water lost acutely, relative to the body weight. A recent weight may be available if the baby has been attending the community clinic and is most helpful as it provides an accurate measurement of fluid loss. One must remember to check though if the clinic weight was without clothes and nappy. The criteria used to assess the degree of dehydration are shown in Figure 2 and listed in Table 3.

An infant who is less than 5% dehydrated does not look unwell. The mucous membranes may be dry but other clinical signs of dehydration are not usually detectable. Beyond 5% dehydration the child looks unwell, the eyes become sunken and in infants the anterior fontanelle is depressed. There is reduction in tissue turgor which is reflected by a decrease in the elasticity of the skin and subcutaneous tissue. This can be appreciated from the delay in the normally instant recoil seen when a fold of skin is picked up between the fingers and then released. These signs are caused by extracellular fluid loss. There is often an acidosis, which may result in tachypnoea, plus a marked reduction in the frequency and quantity of urine passed. When there is peripheral circulatory failure with a thready and rapid pulse, low blood pressure, and cold and poorly perfused extremities more than 10% of body weight is likely to have been lost. By this time the child is gravely ill and the level of consciousness may be reduced.

Table 3   Clinical signs of dehydration

Body weight lost %	Severity	Clinical state	Signs
<5	Mild	Not unwell	Dry mucous membranes; thirst, slight oliguria
5 to 10	Moderate	Apathetic Unwell	Sunken eyes; sunken fontanelle in infants; reduced tissue elasticity; tachypnoea; oliguria
10	Severe	Shocked	Peripheral circulatory failure: hypotension; peripheral vasoconstriction, tachycardia
15	Critical	Moribund	Severely shocked

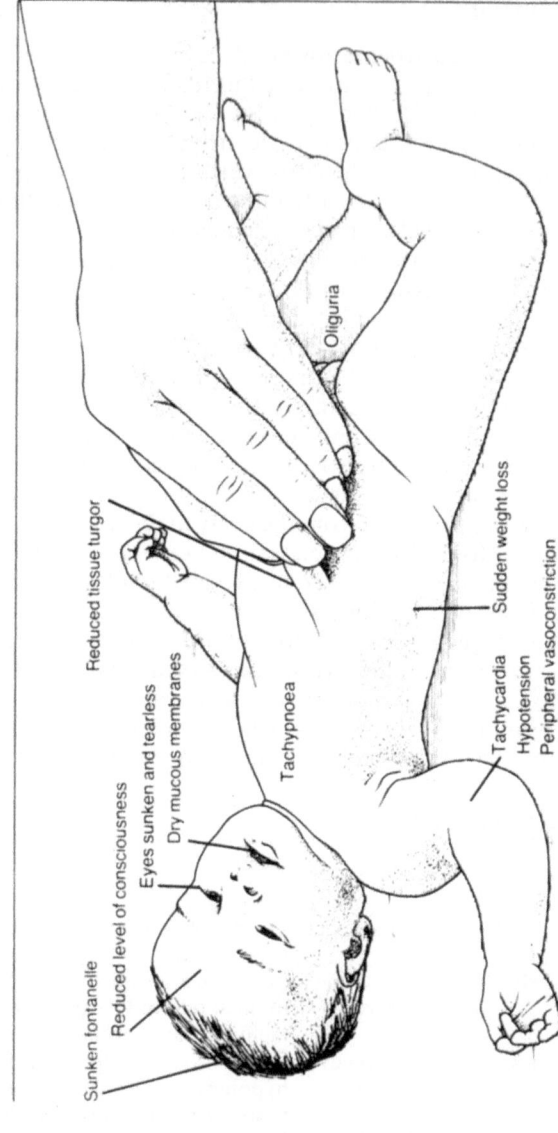

Figure 2 *Clinical features of a severely dehydrated infant with isotonic or hyponatraemic dehydration*

The clinical features of dehydration just described occur when the plasma sodium level is within the normal range, which is the usual finding. If there is hypernatraemia the degree of dehydration may be seriously under-estimated. Other circumstances in which problems arise are the chubby child who may be more dehydrated than he appears, or the malnourished child whose subcutaneous tissue is markedly reduced, also causing sunken eyes and reduced tissue elasticity (Figure 3).

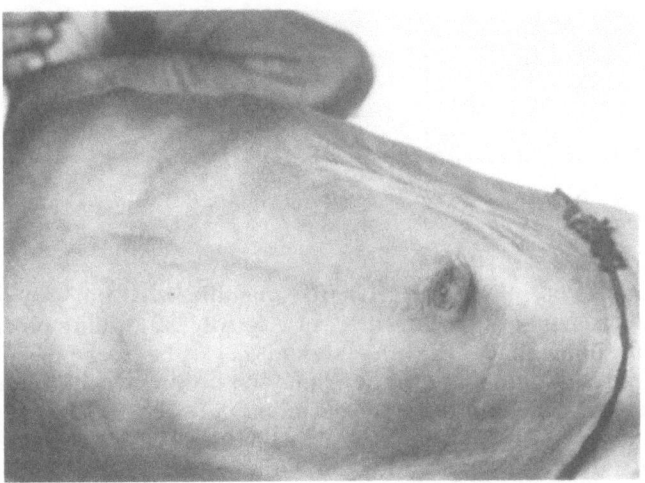

Figure 3   *Delayed recoil of skin from reduced tissue elasticity; this may be found in dehydration or malnutrition*

Oral rehydration

The majority of children can be managed as outpatients. The customary regimen for an infant with gastroenteritis who is mildly dehydrated is to withdraw all milk and solid food from the diet and substitute a solution containing glucose and electrolytes. A glucose-electrolyte mixture (Dioralyte) is now available in sachets and can be simply and accurately made up at home (Figure 4). A less satisfactory, but safe, alternative is to use the fluid from a 0.18% NaCl/4.2% dextrose intravenous infusion. Other solutions such as glucose (three teaspoons added to 200 ml of water), or Coca-Cola

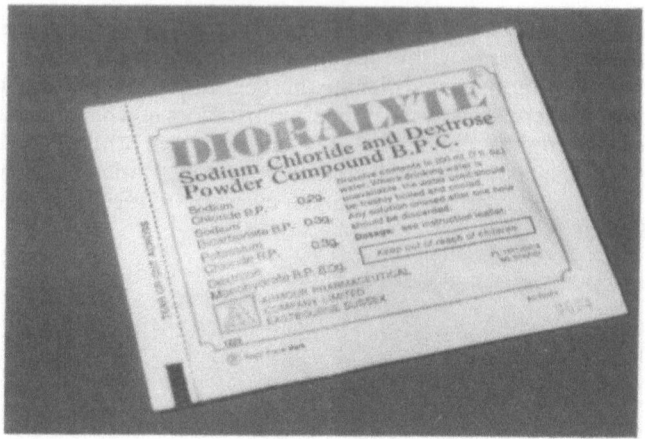

Figure 4   *Sachets of a glucose electrolyte mixture (Dioralyte) which can be safely made up at home*

(which has been left to go flat) are sometimes used but they do not contain adequate concentrations of electrolytes. Adding pinches of salt to home-made mixtures should never be recommended as dangerously high concentrations may be produced with disastrous consequences. Vomiting may be reduced by giving the fluid frequently and in small volumes. After 24 hours of clear fluids, milk can be introduced gradually, starting with a quarter-strength solution and slowly increasing the proportion of milk (Figure 5). At least 150 to 200 ml fluid kg^{-1} $(24 h)^{-1}$ should be given. Toddlers, whose diet is no longer based on milk, can be regraded onto suitable solid foods such as bread, chicken, apples, rice and bananas. Milk or products containing a lot of milk can be avoided until the diarrhoea has settled in case lactose cannot be fully digested and absorbed. As well as discussing the management with the parents, the scheme should be written down in detail. Parents should be warned that their children will need to be seen again if the diarrhoea does not improve, if the fluid intake is insufficient or if symptoms recur when milk or solids are reintroduced.

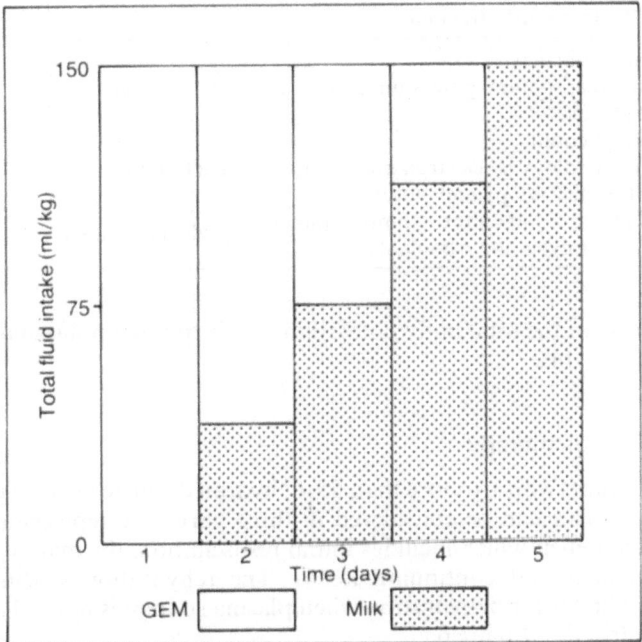

Figure 5 *Oral regrading scheme for infants. GEM = glucose-electrolyte mixture (Dioralyte). Its composition is: sodium 35 mmol/l; potassium 20 mmol/l; chloride 37 mmol/l; bicarbonate 18 mmol/l; dextrose 200 mmol/l or 4 g/100 ml. There are five sachets per litre*

Hospital management

Admission to hospital will be required for children who are more than 5% dehydrated or if the parent is having difficulty dealing with the problem at home. On admission the child's weight must be carefully measured. If an intravenous infusion is started the child should be reweighed with the drip and the splint so that serial measurements can be made. The initial investigations needed are listed in Table 4, and these, together with the clinical assessment, will determine the therapy required. The plasma sodium will reveal whether there is hypernatraemia (Na > 150 mmol/1), normal levels, or hyponatraemia (Na < 130 mmol/l). In almost all cases there is

85

Table 4   Initial investigations

Weight and height
Plasma urea, sodium, potassium and bicarbonate—*urgent*
Blood glucose
Full blood count
Stool for virology by electron microscopy and bacteriology
Urine for microscopy and culture
Blood gases, blood cultures, lumbar puncture $\Big\}$ when indicated
Urine electrolytes and osmolality

depletion of the total body potassium but the plasma potassium may not reflect this.

Intravenous therapy

Most infants who are more than 5% dehydrated will need intravenous therapy. This can be considered in three parts: the replacement of the fluid deficit which includes initial resuscitation, the maintenance requirement and continuing losses. The rehydration scheme described first is for dehydration when plasma sodium is normal and is summarized in Figure 6.

If the infant is shocked, initial resuscitation should be given with 0.9% saline, or a plasma volume expander such as purified plasma fraction in severe cases, giving 10 to 20 ml/kg rapidly. The management of shock is described in more detail in Chapter 11. The remainder of the deficit can be replaced as 0.45% saline/2.5% dextrose. (This solution contains sufficient sodium and chloride to replace the infant's losses as well as providing adequate free water.) The maintenance requirements for the next 24 hours can be calculated from the body weight or surface area (Table 5). Additional fluids may have to be given for continuing losses from fever, hyperventilation or diarrhoea. Once a satisfactory urine output is obtained, potassium chloride (10 to 30 mmol/l) should be added to the infusion. The absence of an adequate urine output following resuscitation may be the result of insufficient fluid replacement or renal insufficiency (see page 198). An eight-month-old infant who was admitted severely dehydrated is shown in Figure 7 together with a regimen for his rehydration.

All children requiring intravenous therapy must be repeatedly

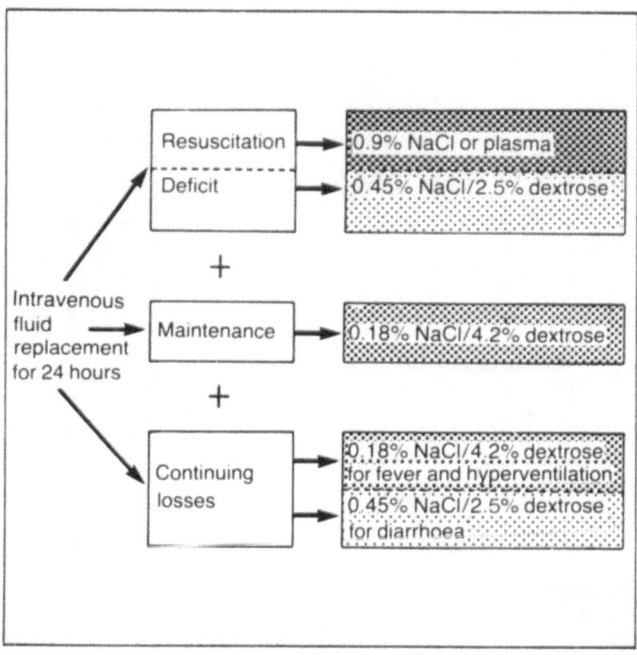

Figure 6 *Summary of intravenous rehydration regimen for infants with a normal plasma sodium*

Table 5 Maintenance intravenous fluid and electrolyte requirements

	Fluid (ml kg⁻¹ (24 h)⁻¹)	Sodium (mmol kg⁻¹ (24 h)⁻¹)	Potassium (mmol kg⁻¹ (24 h)⁻¹)
Body weight			
< 5 kg	150	3.0	3.0
5 to 10 kg	120	3.0	3.0
10 to 20 kg	100	2.5	2.5
> 20 kg	80	2.0	2.0
Surface area	1500 to 2000 ml/m²	50 to 70 mmol/m²	50 to 70 mmol/m²

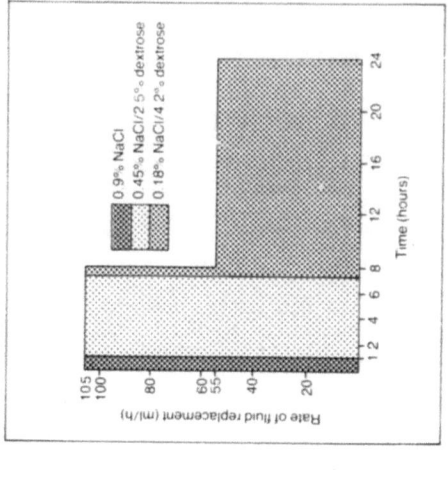

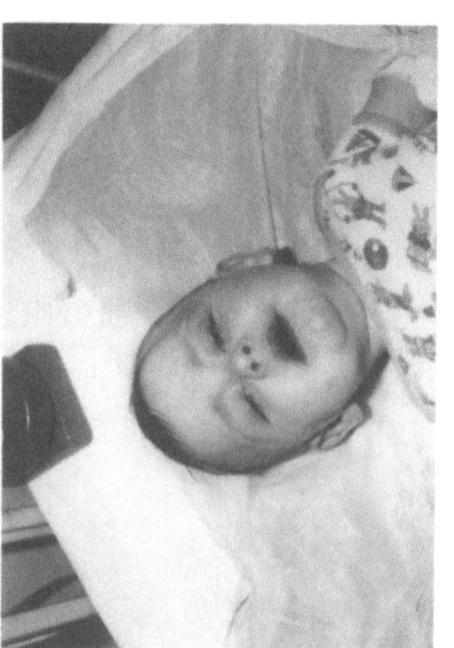

Figure 7a This eight-month-old infant was admitted severely dehydrated with gastroenteritis. Assessment showed 10% dehydration, with a temperature of 39.5°C. He was normonatraemic and weighed 8 kg. **b.** Calculation of the intravenous rehydration regimen used for his treatment. Half the deficit was given in the first eight hours (840 ml at 105 ml/h) and the remainder in the subsequent 16 hours (840 ml at 55 ml/h). Potassium chloride (20 mmol/l) was added after three hours when he had a good urine output. **c.** Breakdown showing the different types of fluid used for rehydration and the rates at which they were given

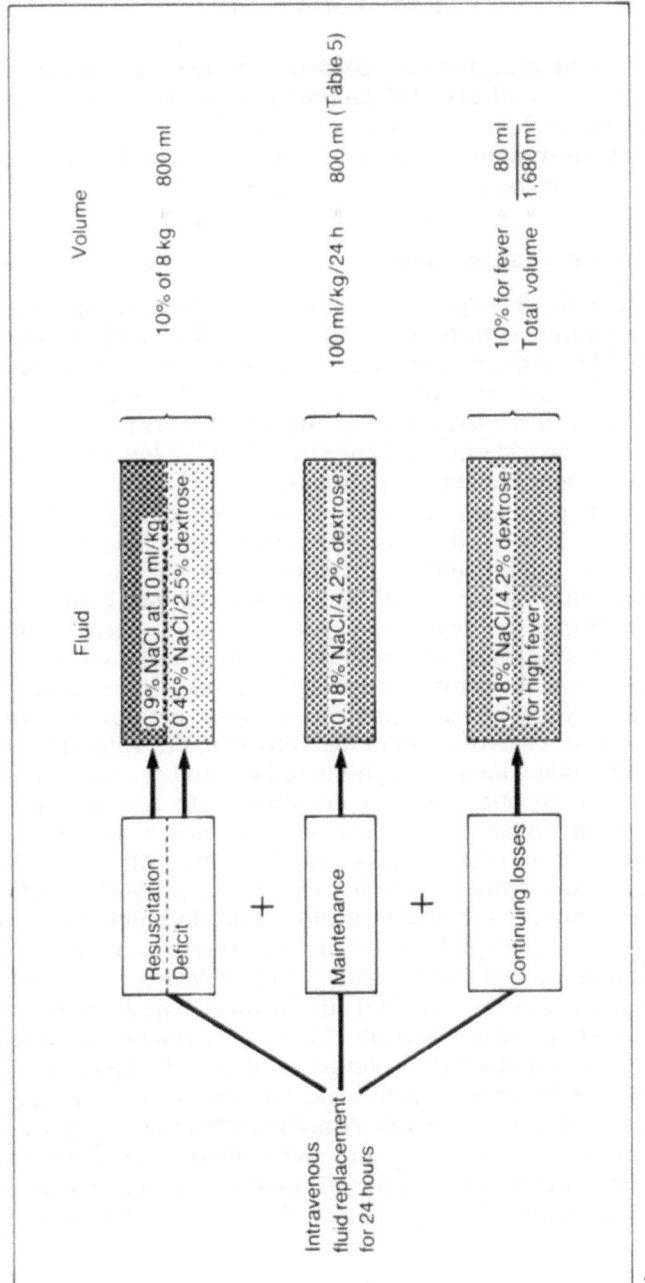

Fluid | Volume

Intravenous fluid replacement for 24 hours

Resuscitation
Deficit — 0.9% NaCl at 10 ml/kg / 0.45% NaCl/2.5% dextrose — 10% of 8 kg = 800 ml

+

Maintenance — 0.18% NaCl/4.2% dextrose — 100 ml/kg/24 h = 800 ml (Table 5)

+

Continuing losses — 0.18% NaCl/4.2% dextrose for high fever — 10% for fever = 80 ml
Total volume = 1,680 ml

b

assessed, and investigations repeated as indicated. The fluid therapy may need to be recalculated if continuing losses from diarrhoea or fever prove to be different from those originally estimated. After 12–24 hours of intravenous rehydration, oral glucose-electrolyte mixture can usually be introduced.

Hypernatraemic dehydration

Hypernatraemic dehydration usually results when an infant with diarrhoea continues to be fed with a high-solute milk. It will be aggravated by fever and hyperventilation which increase insensible water loss. The incidence of hypernatraemic dehydration has fallen dramatically over the last few years and this appears in part to have accompanied the widespread change from high- to low-solute infant milk (Manuel and Walker-Smith, 1980).

When there is an increase in the plasma sodium, an osmotic gradient develops between the intracellular and extracellular fluid compartments. As cell membranes are more permeable to water than ions, water will be drawn out of cells and they will shrink. Intracellular dehydration of cells within the central nervous system results in neurological symptoms, and cerebral vessels may be stretched or torn. In contrast, the peripheral circulation is relatively spared.

The clinical features can be predicted from the pathophysiological changes—central nervous system signs predominate, with a lethargic but irritable child who has a high-pitched cry and gives an exaggerated response to stimulation. Convulsions are not uncommon. Because the peripheral circulation is maintained, even severe dehydration can be difficult to appreciate clinically. Although the skin keeps its turgor, it may feel rather like 'rubbery dough'. There is usually a pronounced metabolic acidosis and the child hyperventilates. It is only when dehydration is very severe and the child is critically ill that peripheral circulatory failure develops. The aim of intravenous therapy is to rehydrate the infant slowly, avoiding rapid changes in extracellular osmolality. Cerebral oedema results if rehydration is too rapid or the solution used is too hypotonic, and convulsions and long-term neurological damage can occur. The rehydration schedule previously described must be modified so that the fluid deficit is corrected slowly and uniformly over 48 hours. Only the initial resuscitation for peripheral circulatory failure will need to be given rapidly, using 0.9% saline or plasma. There is controversy about which solution should be used to replace the remainder of the deficit, but 0.45% NaCl/2.5% dextrose has the advantage of avoiding rapid changes of osmolality. Although the infant will receive more sodium than required, it will be excreted if given slowly. These infants may be severely acidotic, mildly hyperglycaemic and hypocalcaemic and these parameters must be monitored.

Hyponatraemic dehydration

In contrast to infants with hypernatraemic dehydration these children have particularly marked extracellular fluid loss. As a result the clinical signs of dehydration are pronounced and visible early, and are rapidly followed by a fall in plasma volume with circulatory insufficiency. An adequate peripheral circulation must be rapidly re-established with 0.9% saline or plasma. A similar rehydration scheme may be then used as described for normonatraemic dehydration (Figure 6) but the 0.45% NaCl/2.5% dextrose may need to be continued for a longer period. The probable sodium deficit can be calculated from the formula:

$$Na \text{ deficit} = (135 - \text{plasma Na}) \times 0.6$$

where 135 is the desired plasma Na concentration and 0.6 the estimated total body water. Table 6 shows the average electrolyte deficit found in infants who are 10% dehydrated.

Table 6 **Probable deficit in infants with severe dehydration (10%) per kg body weight**

	H_2O (ml)	Na (mmol)	K (mmol)
Isotonic	100	8 to 10	8 to 10
Hypertonic	100	2 to 4	0 to 4
Hypotonic	100	10 to 12	8 to 10

Antiemetic and antidiarrhoeal agents

There is no place for antiemetic and antidiarrhoeal agents in the management of infants with gastroenteritis. There is no evidence that kaolin and pectin, diphenoxylate (Lomotil), or other agents are effective in infants. Diphenoxylate (Lomotil) should never be prescribed for infants as it is particularly dangerous if taken in overdosage, and phenothiazines (such as Stemetil or Maxolon) as antiemetics are best avoided in young children as they are prone to cause dystonic reactions.

Antibiotics

Antibiotics have little place in the routine management of infants with gastroenteritis as the aetiology is usually viral. Even when bacterial pathogens are isolated there is little evidence that antibiotics influence the natural history of the disease or prevent its spread, and there is the danger that they may sometimes prolong the carrier state as in *Salmonella* infections. If there is evidence of septicaemia in association with bacterial gastroenteritis, intravenous antibiotics should be given. They are not required in uncomplicated cases without septicaemia. Most cases of *Campylobacter* infection resolve without any antibiotic therapy. Should an antibiotic be indicated, in vitro studies suggest that most *Campylobacter* are sensitive to erythromycin.

Isolation

Infants with diarrhoea should be barrier nursed with diligent hand washing and the use of gowns to prevent spread to other children. Disposable gloves are advisable when nappies are changed.

To be confined to an isolation cubicle is inevitably unpleasant, but this may be reduced to a minimum if everyone concerned is aware of the problem. The child's mother should be encouraged to be resident, and suitable toys and a television provided.

Recurrence of symptoms

Recurrence of symptoms during regrading may arise from an acute and transient intolerance to the increased strength of milk. This is usually caused by lactose intolerance which results from damage to the most superficial part of the villi in the brush border of the small intestine, where lactase is normally found. The stool will contain unaltered lactose and as this is a reducing substance it can be detected with a Clinitest tablet (adding five drops of stool supernatant and 10 drops of water) which is positive if there is more than 0.5% reducing substance present. Even if lactose can be digested into monosaccharides, the absorption of the monosaccharides may be impaired and they may emerge in the stool and will also be detected on testing for reducing substances. This acquired lactose intolerance may be associated with cows' milk protein intolerance.

Infants who relapse when milk is reintroduced can often be managed by a return to clear fluids and then regraded onto milk again. Even if this fails, the problem is usually transient and may be managed by substituting for a few weeks a milk which contains neither lactose nor cows' milk protein. Occasionally, the problem becomes chronic with persistent diarrhoea and failure to thrive.

Vomiting

Many babies regurgitate part of their feed. If this is frequent parents may become concerned and also exasperated by the constant dribbling of milk over themselves and their household. This is most often because of gastro-oesophageal reflux through a lax lower oesophageal sphincter. If the baby is perfectly healthy, is gaining weight and growth is satisfactory, sympathetic reassurance or some symptomatic help is all that is required. The problem mostly disappears at about a year of age when the child starts to be on his feet.

If the vomiting is more severe the baby may fail to thrive and further investigation will be indicated. A barium swallow is the simplest and most informative test. It may show reflux of barium and there may be a co-existing hiatus hernia. Ulceration of the oesophagus from persistent reflux may result in blood staining of the vomit and anaemia. Complications which have been ascribed to gastro-oesophageal reflux include stricture formation of the lower oesophagus and respiratory symptoms including apnoea, pneumonia or wheezing from recurrent aspiration.

Medical management is mainly symptomatic, by nursing the infant upright in a chair, thickening the milk and sometimes with antacids (for example with Infant Gaviscon). Further investigation and rarely surgical repair with fundal plication will need to be considered when medical treatment fails or for life-threatening complications. Other important causes of vomiting in a well baby are incorrect feeding techniques or problems in the relationship between the mother and her baby.

The causes of vomiting in infancy are numerous and the important causes have been listed in Table 7. If the infant is ill or the vomiting

Table 7   Some important causes of vomiting in infants

Feeding problems
Gastroenteritis
Infections:
   Respiratory tract infection
   Otitis media
   Urinary tract infection
   Septicaemia, meningitis
Intestinal obstruction, e.g. pyloric stenosis and intussusception
Gastro-oesophageal reflux (hiatus hernia)
Food allergy
Raised intracranial pressure
Drugs
Renal insufficiency
Congenital adrenal hyperplasia
Inborn errors of metabolism

of acute onset the cause will need to be assessed immediately. Any infections will need to be identified, surgical conditions in particular pyloric stenosis, intussusception and other forms of intestinal obstruction and appendicitis and peritonitis excluded. Rarely the infant will have congenital adrenal hyperplasia, renal failure or an inherited metabolic disorder.

Infections

In contrast to adults, almost any infection of infancy may present with vomiting, even in the absence of fever. In addition to gastroenteritis some of the more important infections to consider are upper and lower respiratory tract infections, otitis media, urinary tract infection, osteomyelitis, septicaemia and meningitis.

Pyloric stenosis

Babies with pyloric stenosis mostly present between three and eight weeks of age with a history of intermittent vomiting which occurs especially after feeds, is effortless, copious and projectile. Afterwards the baby is hungry and wants another feed. Pyloric stenosis is more common in boys, in first-born babies and there may be a family history. It is found in preterm infants, and pyloric stenosis has been

94

seen in infants weighing less than 1 kg. The longer the delay in diagnosis the more dehydrated and malnourished the child will be.

In most cases the diagnosis can be confirmed during a test feed. The infant should be fed at the mother's left breast or held so that the baby's head is on her left side if bottle-fed. During the feed or shortly afterwards the pylorus contracts and can then be palpated. It lies under the right rectus muscle and feels like an olive. It can best be palpated by cupping the fingers over and under the lateral margin of the right rectus. If a pyloric mass cannot be felt on the first occasion the feed may need to be repeated. It may be difficult to feel if the stomach is distended and initial aspiration of the gastric contents may help. Waves of peristalsis of the stomach wall may be visible travelling from left to right across the epigastrium but this can also be seen in some normal infants and undue reliance should not be placed on this sign alone. Occasionally, a diagnosis cannot be made in this way and an ultrasound or barium meal may be necessary.

The treatment for pyloric stenosis is Ramstedt's operation where the hypertrophied muscle is incised taking care not to perforate the mucosa. If the plasma electrolytes or bicarbonate concentration are abnormal or the baby is clinically dehydrated initial intravenous rehydration will be required. Characteristically, there is a hypochloraemic alkalosis and a marked depletion of the intracellular potassium. The plasma potassium is also usually low. Initial rehydration can be with 0.9% NaCl, 10 to 20 ml/kg, followed by 0.45% NaCl/2.5% dextrose with added potassium chloride until the fluid deficit has been replaced.

Intestinal obstruction

Intestinal obstruction in the first few months is most frequently caused by congenital abnormalities such as intestinal atresia or stenosis, malrotation or Hirschsprung's disease. The more proximal the obstruction the more prominent the vomiting, and whenever bile is present in vomit it should be assumed to be caused by intestinal obstruction until proved otherwise (Figure 8). As the obstruction becomes more distal, vomiting will occur later but abdominal distension will become more pronounced (Figure 9). In infants, intussusception is the most common cause of intestinal obstruction, with a

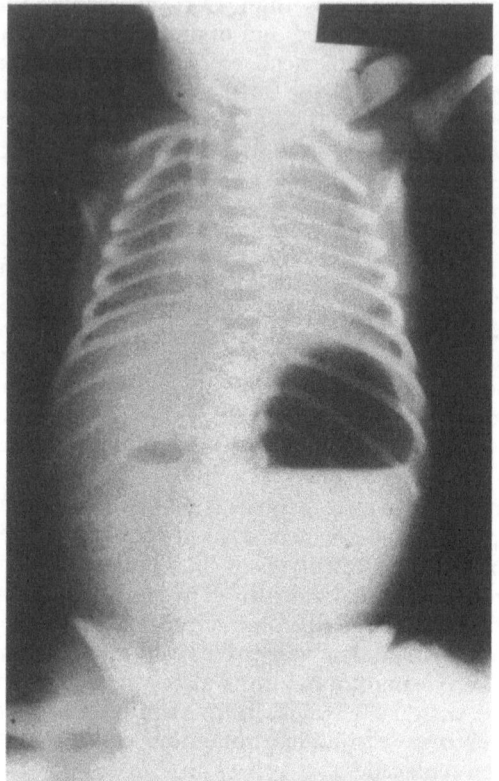

Figure 8   *Duodenal atresia showing the characteristic 'double bubble' appearance in the erect abdominal radiograph. There is air in the stomach and proximal duodenum but none beyond the obstruction*

peak incidence between six and twelve months. Strangulated inguinal hernias occur at all ages.

Congenital adrenal hyperplasia

Females with congenital adrenal hyperplasia are usually identified at birth because of masculinization of the external genitalia (Figure 10). Unless there is a family history males with this condition are rarely

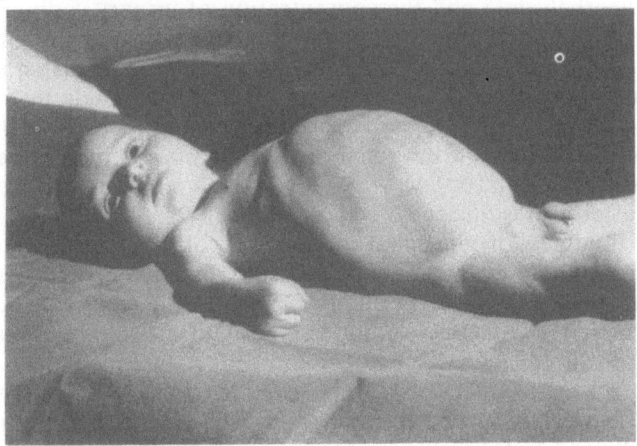

Figure 9 *Gross abdominal distension in a two-month-old infant with Hirschsprung's disease*

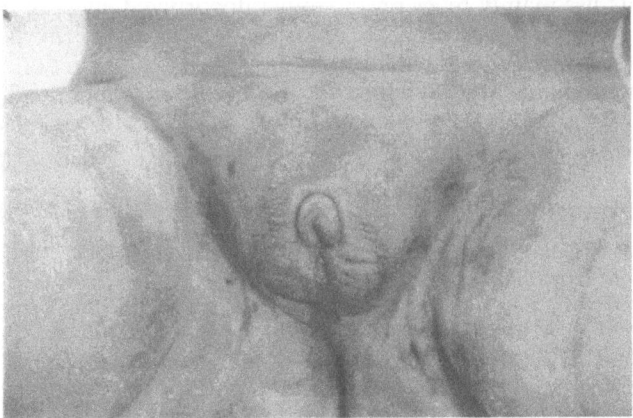

Figure 10 *External genitalia of a female infant with congenital adrenal hyperplasia. There is enlargement of the clitoris and the labia are fused*

identified at birth. Between 30 and 50% of these infants are salt-losers and may present at 10 to 14 days of age or earlier with vomiting and some diarrhoea. If their condition is not recognized early they may become shocked. Serum electrolytes show marked hyponatraemia and hyperkalaemia and the concentration of urinary sodium is inappropriately high. Hyponatraemia is most commonly the result of excessive loss of sodium into the gut from vomiting or diarrhoea. In sodium losing states the urine sodium is inappropriately high compared with the plasma sodium concentration and the sodium intake. When the salt loss is from renal disease the plasma potassium concentration is normal or low, whilst hyperkalaemia is a notable feature of aldosterone insufficiency.

The treatment of congenital adrenal hyperplasia comprises sodium replacement and giving mineralocorticoids and glucocorticoids. Immediate management of an infant in a salt losing crisis is to administer salt and re-expand the blood volume with 0.9% saline or plasma. Dextrose should be added to the infusion if the infant has a low blood glucose. Mineralocorticoid (deoxycortone pivalate (Percorten-M)) is often needed in infants and the response is monitored clinically and by following the blood pressure and plasma and urine electrolytes. Hydrocortisone (50-100 mg) is rarely required in the emergency situation unless the child is severely shocked and even then its use mainly relies on the mineralocorticoid effect of cortisol which is poor compared to aldosterone. In 21-hydroxylase deficiency, which is by far the commonest form, the secretion rate of cortisol remains normal whilst the ACTH drive is high, and giving hydrocortisone makes it much more difficult to establish the diagnosis.

References

Barnes, N.D. and Roberton, N.R.C. (1979), *Update*, **18,** 885.
Br. Med. J., leading article, 1980, **281,** 1162.
Lewis, H.M., Parry, J.V., Davies, H.A., Parry, R.P., Sanderson, P.J., Tyrrell, D.A. and Valman, H.B., (1979), *Arch. Dis. Child.*, **54,** 339.
Manuel, P.D. and Walker-Smith, J.A., (1980), *Arch. Dis. Child.*, **55,** 124.

Further reading

Brook, C.G.D., (1978), *Practical Paediatric Endocrinology*, Academic Press, London.
Harris, F.(1972), *Paediatric Fluid Therapy*, Blackwell Scientific Publications, London.
Houston, I.B. (1978), Fluid and electrolytes, in *Clinical Paediatric Physiology*, Godfrey, S. and Baum, J.D. (Eds.), Blackwell Scientific Publications, London.

Valman, H.B. (1979), Gastroenteritis, in *Paediatric Therapeutics*, Valman, H.B. (Ed.), Blackwell Scientific Publications, London.

Walker-Smith, J.A. (1979), *Diseases of the Small Intestine in Childhood*, Pitman Medical, Tunbridge Wells.

Winters, R.W. (Ed.) (1973), *The Body Fluids in Pediatrics*, Little, Brown & Co., Boston.

CHAPTER 6

Acute abdominal pain

Children frequently complain of abdominal pain. However, as young children find it more difficult to localize pain than adults, it is important not to confine one's attention to the abdomen, but to consider the whole child. It is then possible to decide whether the source of pain is within or outside the abdomen. Extensive lists can be made of the possible causes of acute abdominal pain in children but these tend to confuse the situation by burying the common among the obscure. A more pragmatic approach will be adopted in this chapter. Some of the more common causes are listed in Figure 1.

Extra-abdominal causes

Referred abdominal pain may be caused by infections of the upper and lower respiratory tract, for example tonsillitis, otitis media or pneumonia. Lower lobe pneumonia may sometimes be detected on auscultation, but it may be evident only on a chest radiograph. An important clue to this diagnosis is the respiratory rate, which is invariably raised in children with pneumonia. Young children with a strangulated inguinal hernia or torsion of the testis may only indicate a painful abdomen, and the hernial orifices and genitalia need to be examined carefully at all ages.

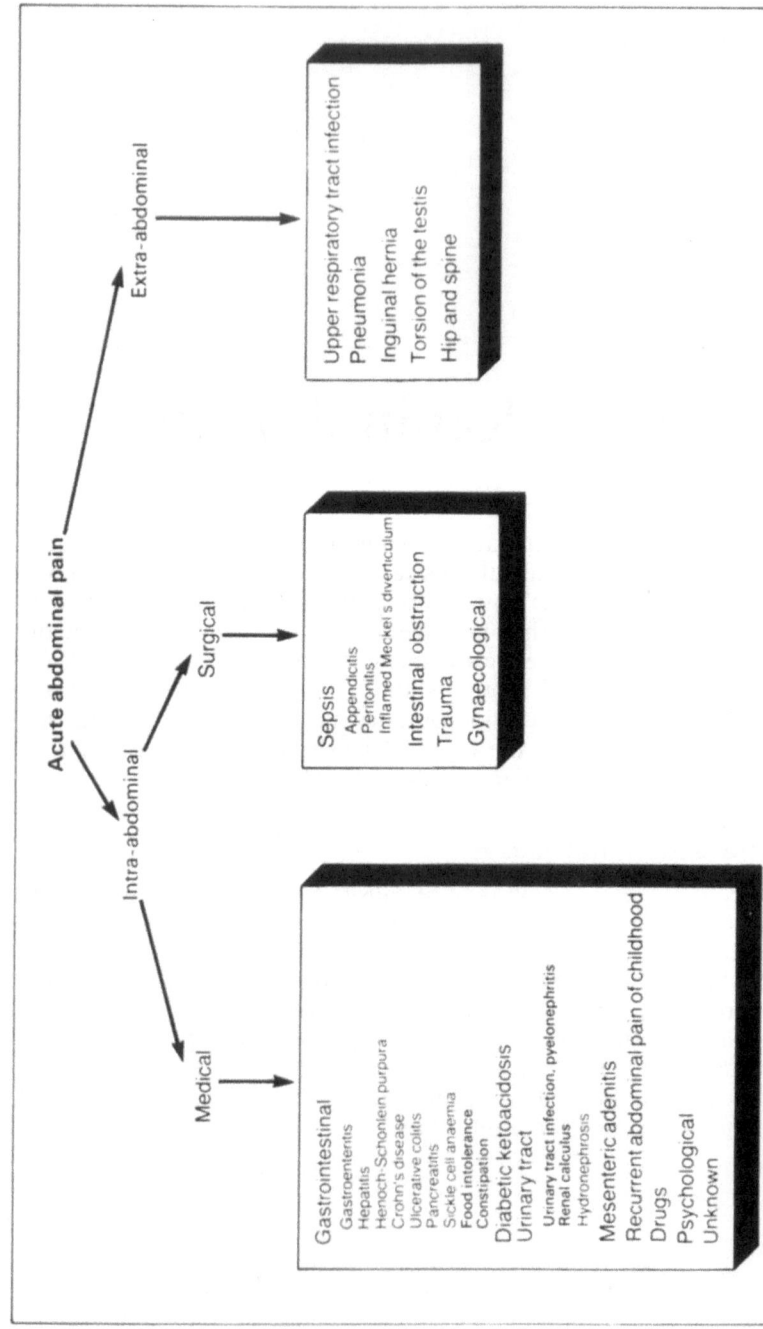

Figure 1 *Important causes of acute abdominal pain in childhood*

Age less than two years

In children less than two years, abdominal pain is frequently associated with intestinal obstruction. Intussusception and a strangulated inguinal hernia are the most important causes, being more frequent than appendicitis in this age group. Malrotation and volvulus are rarer causes of obstruction. The serious causes of acute abdominal pain in this age group are listed in Table 1.

Table 1   Serious causes of acute abdominal pain in infants less than two years old

Intestinal obstruction:
    Intussusception
    Strangulated inguinal hernia
    Malrotation and volvulus
Appendicitis

Intussusception

The peak incidence of intussusception is between six and twelve months of age and the commonest site is the terminal ileum or the ileocaecal valve, resulting in an ileocolic intussusception. The classical features are colicky abdominal pain, vomiting, the passage of blood-stained stools and the presence of an abdominal mass. The characteristic history is of a previously well infant who suddenly develops paroxysms of screaming, with his legs drawn up onto the abdomen. The intensity of the crying and the accompanying pallor usually leave the parents in no doubt that their child is in pain. The attacks last for a minute or two, and recur at intervals of 15 to 30 minutes. Initially the infant will play and appear his usual self between attacks, but later he remains pale, clammy and exhausted between spasms. Vomiting usually follows, as does constipation, although one or two loose stools may be passed initially. The passage of blood and mucus per rectum, the well known 'red currant jelly' stools, are a late feature and may be detected only when a rectal examination is done.

The intussusception may be palpable as a sausage-shaped mass when the child is relaxed between bouts of colic, usually in the right upper quadrant (Figure 2). It may be particularly difficult to feel when it lies under the liver edge and may require deep palpation to

103

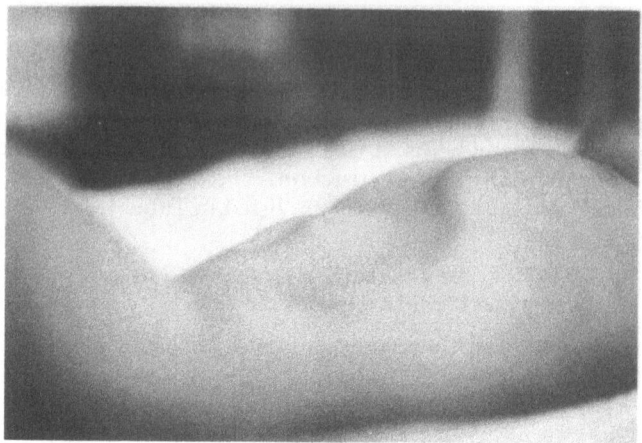

Figure 2   *The mass from an intussusception is visible in this dehydrated and thin child*

be appreciated. Occasionally it may only be palpable with the tip of a finger on rectal examination. Unfortunately, the classical features are not always present and the child tends to pay for this with a delay in the diagnosis. Intussusception may be painless in as many as 10% of cases, and these infants may present in shock before the diagnosis is made. In others, vomiting may be absent, particularly if the intussusception is located in the large bowel, and not infrequently the characteristic blood-stained stools are absent. A mass is not palpable in a third of cases.

The diagnosis is usually made clinically by the combination of the history, observation and palpation of the intussusception, but in cases of doubt radiography will be needed. A straight abdominal radiograph may show the head of the intussusception as a soft tissue mass outlined by air lying distal to the obstruction. If it is ileocaecal, there may be an absence of gas in the right iliac fossa and distended loops of small intestine. A barium enema can be used both to confirm the diagnosis and as a therapeutic procedure to attempt to reduce the intussusception by hydrostatic pressure (Figure 3). In many centres it has become the treatment of choice for early uncomplicated cases. It can only be used if an experienced radiologist is immediately available, as any delay in treatment increases the risk of complica-

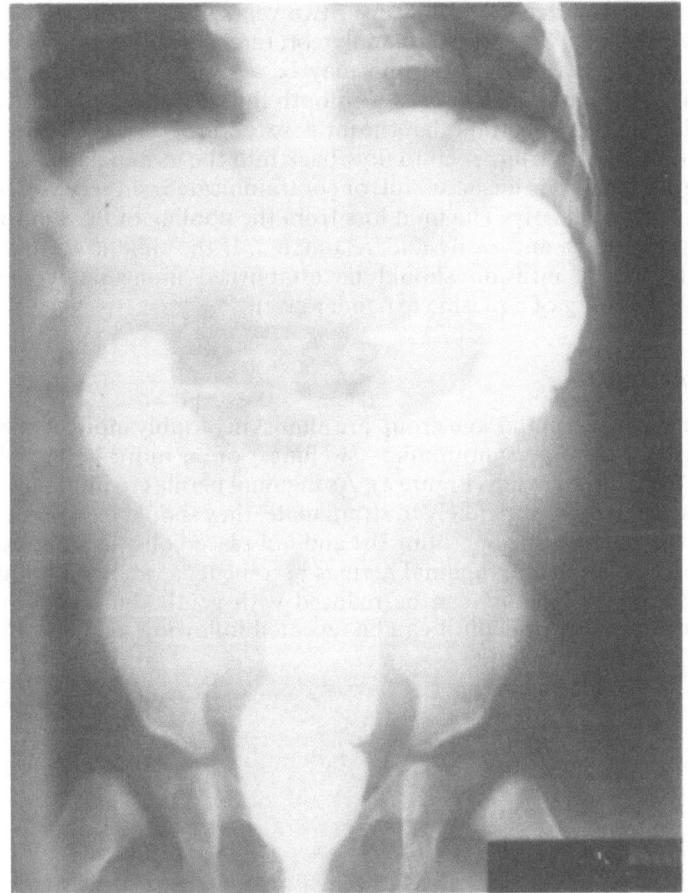

Figure 3 *A barium enema in an eight-month-old child, demonstrating an intussusception preventing the proximal flow of barium. It was successfully reduced with the barium enema*

tions and is unpleasant for the child. The danger of this conservative approach is the possible reduction of non-viable or gangrenous bowel with the risk of perforation and it is definitely contraindicated if the child is toxic and in need of resuscitation. It is also advisable to exclude those with a history longer than 24 hours and those outside the typical age range. The child over two years of age is more likely to have a Meckel's diverticulum, polyp or, rarely, a lymphoma at the apex. The reduction with barium may be assisted by giving intravenous glucagon, which acts as a smooth muscle relaxant, and the radiologist must be certain that the intussusception has been reduced completely with barium seen to flow back into the terminal ileum. If the barium enema is unsuccessful, or contraindicated, surgery will be required immediately. The fluid loss from the pooling of fluid in the gut is often large and easily underestimated. If the child is at all ill, an intravenous infusion should be established immediately and initially 20 ml/kg of a plasma expander given.

Inguinal hernia

Inguinal hernias in this age group are almost invariably indirect. The majority present as symptomless swellings, often more noticeable when the baby is crying (Figure 4). As inguinal hernias in infants less than a year old are very likely to strangulate, they should be operated on at the next routine operating list and not placed on a waiting list.

When strangulated, inguinal hernias become tense and tender but even at this stage most can be reduced with gentle manipulation; should this prove difficult it can be repeated following sedation and

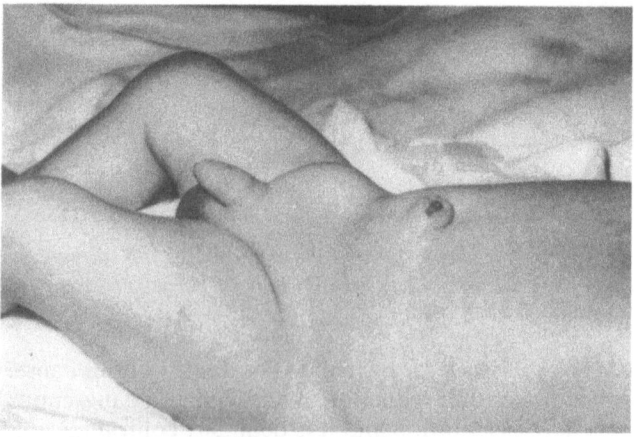

Figure 4 Inguinal hernias in infants less than a year old are very liable to strangulate and should be repaired promptly

elevation of the legs. If the hernia is successfully reduced surgery can be performed 24 to 48 hours later, when the tissue oedema has resolved. If unsuccessful, immediate operation will be necessary.

Malrotation

In the commonest type, instead of the caecum descending *in utero* into the right iliac fossa, it remains in the upper abdomen, lying to the left of the duodenum (Figure 5). Peritoneal bands which fix the caecum to the posterior abdominal wall (Ladd's bands) may cross

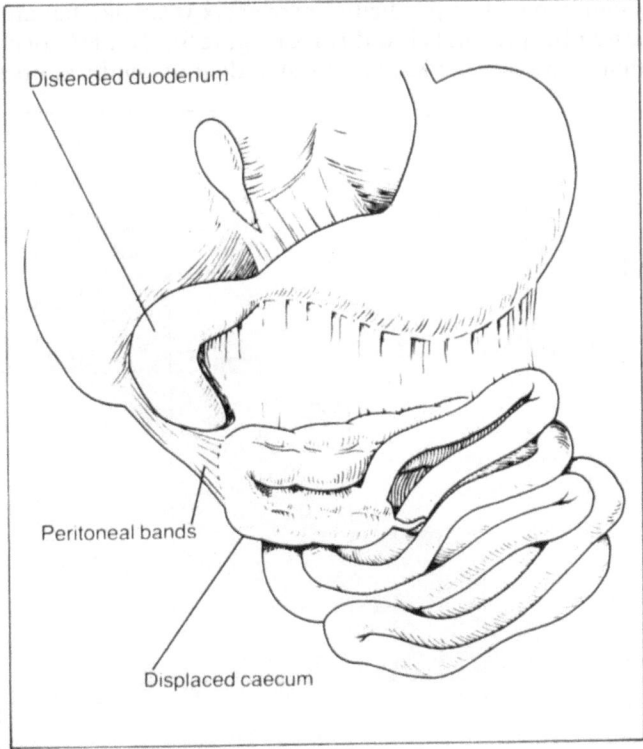

Figure 5 *Malrotation, showing the caecum lying to the left of the duodenum and peritoneal bands crossing anterior to the duodenum. The midgut is prone to volvulus as it is suspended from a narrow pedicle*

anterior to the duodenum and cause incomplete duodenal obstruction. The midgut is suspended from a narrow pedicle which contains the superior mesenteric vessels and is prone to volvulus. With tightening of the volvulus, the mesenteric vessels become occluded and the midgut will become gangrenous unless it is promptly relieved. Although most children with malrotation present with duodenal obstruction in the neonatal period it may present in older children. Symptoms may also be intermittent.

Appendicitis

Most children with appendicitis are over six years old, but an appreciable number present below this age (Figure 6). Over 80% of children less than two years old have perforated their appendix at operation,

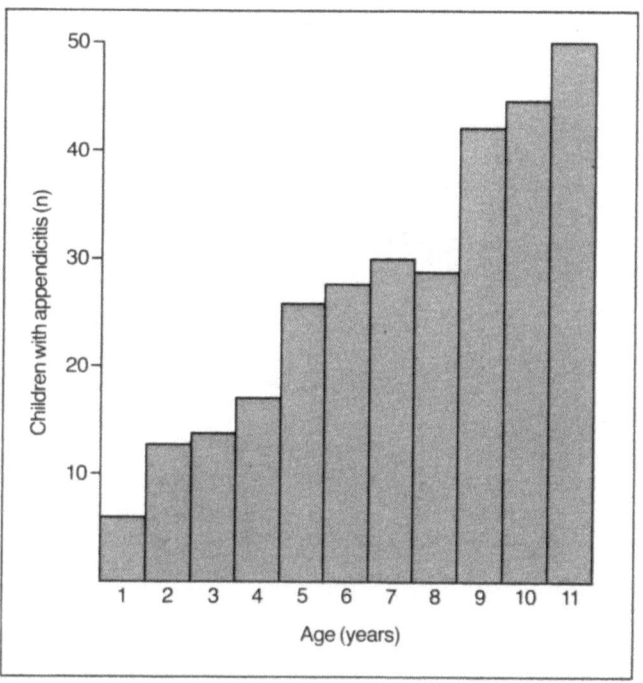

Figure 6 *The age distribution of children with appendicitis. (After Jackson, 1963)*

and there is a high morbidity and appreciable mortality. Common symptoms and signs include vomiting, lethargy and irritability, followed by abdominal distension. Abdominal tenderness is difficult to appreciate in an infant, and the high incidence of perforation is a consequence of late diagnosis.

Age over two years

Young children can provide a more detailed history than an infant, and examination may reveal more specific signs, but these will still be much less precise than an adult can give.

The history will usually be provided by the parent but children should always be offered the opportunity to give their own account too. The same significance cannot be attached to the site of pain in a young child as in an adult or older child. The nature of the pain is also difficult for children to describe and they may need help in verbalizing what they are feeling. The most important information is the duration of the pain and whether it is getting worse or better.

Few toddlers will willingly allow a stranger to feel their tummy, unless they are too ill to object, but with patience most children can be induced to lie down so that a thorough examination can be made. With small children it may help to make an initial examination while they sit on their mother's knee. Small toys or a torch may help distract them while enquiries about school, pets or family will divert older children's attention away from the abdomen. While palpating the abdomen, starting away from the site that is said to be tender, the child's face should be watched to see if he winces or objects. This will usually overcome any confusion from children who agree that they are tender from a desire to please the examiner, or others who are frightened of a stay in hospital or an operation and stoically deny any pain at all on direct questioning. It may also be helpful to palpate the abdomen using the child's own hand.

Sedating a distressed child (with chloral hydrate (Noctec), 30 mg/kg or trimeprazine (Vallergan) 2 to 4 mg/kg) may occasionally be helpful. In children, rectal examination rarely yields information about tenderness which has not been elicited on abdominal palpation. Very occasionally it may enable one to appreciate a pelvic abscess or a mass, and it may be helpful in infants with an intussusception.

Deciding whether or not a child requires surgery is the key decision to be taken when assessing a child with abdominal pain. By far the commonest indication for surgery is, of course, appendicitis, and the reduction in mortality and morbidity from this has largely resulted from its early recognition and prompt surgical treatment. The main difficulty lies in distinguishing children with appendicitis from the even larger group who do not require surgery. The causes of acute abdominal pain in children over two years of age who were admitted to hospital in Southampton during one year are shown in Figure 7.

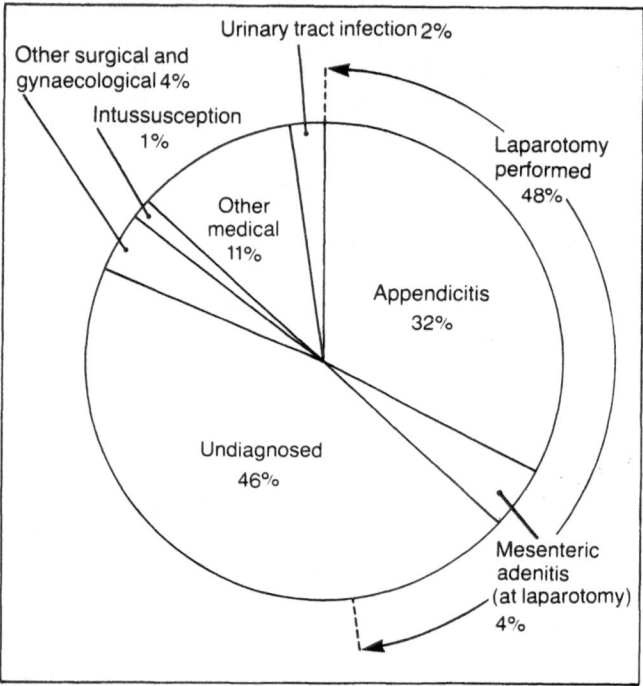

Figure 7 *Causes of acute abdominal pain in children over two years old who were admitted to hospital during the course of one year. Trauma has been excluded. (After Drake, 1980)*

Appendicitis

To avoid delay in the diagnosis of appendicitis, it is generally wise to admit all children with significant abdominal pain lasting longer than four hours. In the older child one may obtain a history of the classical features of intense continuous periumbilical pain moving to the right iliac fossa. Vomiting occurs in over 90% of cases, though it is not persistent or copious. It almost always begins after the onset of the pain, in contrast to gastroenteritis, where the vomiting precedes the pain. Anorexia is almost universal. A low-grade fever is common, but a high fever may be found with perforation or an appendix abscess. These characteristic features may be found when the appendix lies in the classical position, and inflammatory fluid readily comes into contact with the anterior abdominal wall. However, in a large number of children with appendicitis in Newcastle, only 32% were in the classical site, while 27% were retrocaecal, 23% pelvic and the remaining 11% in other sites (retroileal, subhepatic, splenic or left iliac fossa) (Jackson, 1963). This may explain why the typical features are so often absent, and why the diagnosis continues to be such a challenge. Indeed, in this series, the pain began in the right lower quadrant in a quarter of the children, and remained central in a further 25%. Whereas the pain was persistent in most, it was intermittent throughout the illness in 10% and began as intermittent pain but later became persistent in a third.

Abdominal tenderness may be slight or absent when the appendix is retrocaecal, retroileal or pelvic, but steady finger pressure may elicit a deeply placed tender point. In cases where the inflamed appendix is pelvic, urinary symptoms may be prominent. Another pitfall is that there may be diarrhoea rather than the usual mild constipation, so that an initial diagnosis of gastroenteritis is made.

The white blood count is in general unhelpful, showing an increase in neutrophil polymorphs and a left shift only if peritonitis is present. Radiographs are unnecessary in most instances but can be of assistance in problem cases. An empty right iliac fossa with signs of intestinal obstruction is very suggestive, as is the finding of a calcified faecolith. The MSU may show an increase in white cells if the inflamed appendix is retrocaecal or pelvic, or occasionally a urinary tract infection may be a coincidental finding.

When the diagnosis is uncertain, the child should be reassessed clinically at regular and frequent intervals (every one to two hours) so that a working diagnosis can be reached within a few hours.

Mesenteric adenitis

Many of the children who do not have appendicitis are said to have mesenteric adenitis. Many of those in this heterogeneous group have viral infections, and a few have *Yersinia*. Typically they have an upper respiratory tract infection, high fever, lymphadenopathy and a site of maximal abdominal tenderness which migrates and is said to be caused by enlarged mesenteric lymph nodes. It is very informative to re-examine the abdomen of all children with suspected appendicitis or mesenteric adenitis shortly after admission to the ward, as it is not uncommon for there to be a marked alteration in physical signs from the initial assessment in the accident and emergency department.

Peritonitis

Few conditions other than a perforated appendix cause peritonitis in children. Other rarer causes include a perforated Meckel's diverticulum and perforation following intestinal obstruction.

There is usually abdominal distension, but in infants and young children board-like rigidity may not be present. Rather, one sees a flushed, toxic, over-alert child with poor peripheral circulation, who is in danger of sudden collapse from shock. Initial resuscitation with intravenous fluids, nasogastric decompression and broad spectrum antibiotics, such as cephaloridine (Ceporin) and metronidazole (Flagyl) need to be given before surgery.

Meckel's diverticulum

An inflamed Meckel's diverticulum may mimic appendicitis or serve as a focus for intestinal obstruction. It is also an important cause of both acute and chronic gastrointestinal haemorrhage in children. A Meckel's diverticulum can often be identified with a technetium scan by demonstrating the abnormally situated gastric mucosa which usually lines the diverticulum.

Medical causes

Urinary tract

It is imperative that all children with abdominal pain, whether acute or chronic, have a urine specimen examined microscopically and cultured. The importance of diagnosing a urinary tract infection lies not only in establishing the appropriate therapy but also in initiating radiographic investigations and follow-up.

With acute pyelonephritis the diagnosis may be made more difficult by a negative urine culture in the early stages.

With hydronephrosis, the enlarged kidney may be tender and palpable only at times of outflow obstruction (Figure 8).

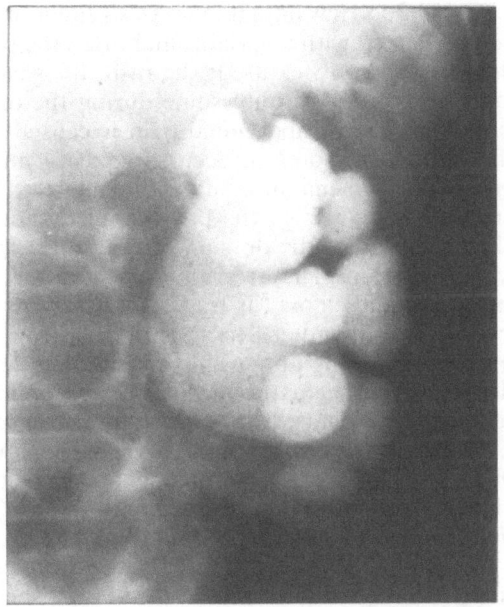

Figure 8   *An intravenous urogram showing unilateral hydronephrosis from a pelviureteric junction obstruction. It had caused left-sided abdominal pain*

Gastrointestinal

Gastroenteritis is often accompanied by abdominal pain and may imitate appendicitis, but normally there is marked diarrhoea and vomiting. There may be some degree of abdominal distension and fluid levels may be present on an abdominal radiograph. *Salmonella* and *Campylobacter* infections are particularly commonly associated with abdominal pain. Hepatitis may also cause pain and tenderness in the right upper quadrant, but the diagnosis may not be clinically obvious in the preicteric phase.

In Henoch-Schönlein purpura, as well as involvement of the skin, there may be gastrointestinal, joint and renal manifestations. It mainly affects the preschool child. The pathognomonic feature is the rash, with its characteristic distribution over the buttocks, lower limbs and elbows (Figure 9). It varies from red macules to papules and purpura with or without ecchymoses, while in the very young, it may be urticarial. After a few days it fades to a yellow-brown colour. The rash occurs in crops with a variable and often relapsing course. Although the most obvious feature is the rash, the gastrointestinal manifestations are the most troublesome during the initial illness. Severe colicky or persistent abdominal pain is caused by haemorrhage into the bowel wall. Vomiting occurs frequently and there may be haematemesis and melaena. Intussusception may develop and can be difficult to differentiate from the pre-existing symptoms. Other features include oedema of the dorsum of the hands and feet and occasionally of the scalp. The arthritis, which mainly affects the ankles, knees, wrists and elbows, is transient. Renal involvement is the most serious problem with a 1 to 3% mortality from glomerulonephritis. On routine testing about half the children develop albuminuria and microscopic haematuria, while macroscopic haematuria is present in a quarter. Those with symptomless proteinuria and haematuria, which may last for months or years, generally do well, but up to 20% may develop permanent renal damage. Altogether the nephritis of Henoch-Schönlein purpura accounts for 15% of children requiring dialysis for end-stage renal failure (Meadow, 1980). No drugs have been shown to affect the progression or recurrence of the acute illness, although it has been claimed that a short course of steroids may reduce the severity of troublesome abdominal pain.

Crohn's disease, ulcerative colitis, peptic ulceration and pancreatitis are all uncommon in children, but their incidence is increasing. Pancreatitis is most often a feature of mumps or trauma. Food intolerance associated with lactose deficiency or true food allergic disorders may present with abdominal pain which may be acute or recurrent. Definitive diagnosis is not easy but a reproducible immediate reaction following ingestion of lactose or a particular food may suggest the diagnosis. Such diagnoses are at present fashionable but conclusive proof is not easily obtained when reactions occur hours or days after ingestion.

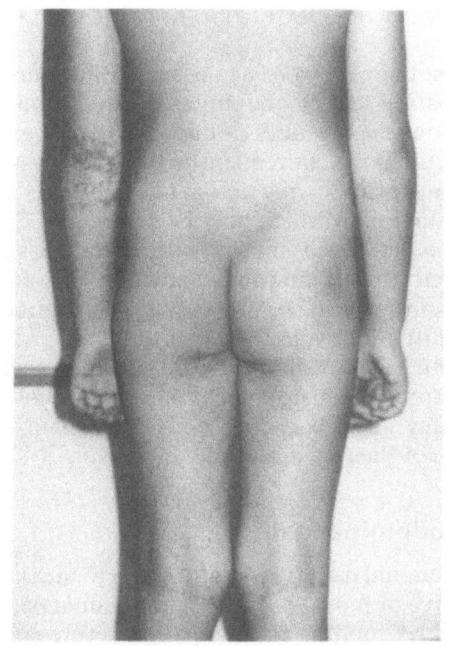

a

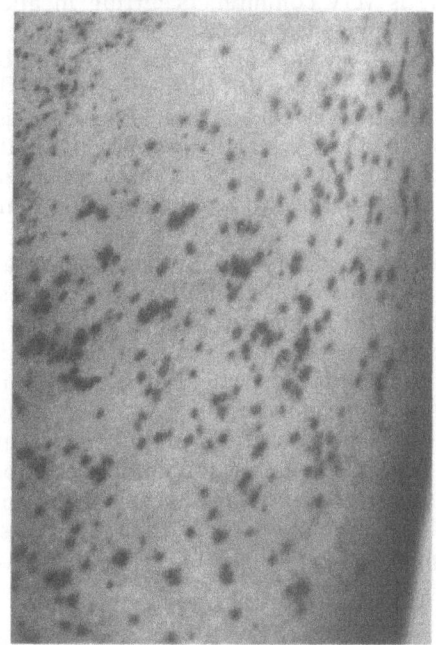

b

Figure 9 *Henoch-Schönlein purpura. (a) Distribution over the buttocks, lower limbs and elbows. (b) Close-up of the typical purpuric and maculopapular rash*

There does not appear to be a consensus of opinion as to whether or not constipation causes abdominal pain. Chronic constipation, even of enormous degree, does not appear to cause pain. However, acute constipation, not infrequently from excessive use of anti-diarrhoeal agents or following an anal fissure, does appear to cause colicky abdominal pain which may be severe and disappears when the constipation is relieved. Infants with an anal fissure may scream on opening their bowels, and may show obvious anxiety in anticipation of the painful event. Laxatives may be required to ensure that the stools are soft and to allow the fissure to heal.

Children with sickle cell disease may suffer severe abdominal pain from infarction during a sickling crisis. Those with diabetic ketoacidosis may also experience abdominal pain, which resolves with correction of their metabolic derangement.

Recurrent abdominal pain

Recurrent abdominal pain is generally taken to mean that a child has experienced three or more episodes of abdominal pain over a period of more than three months and the pain is severe enough to restrict his activities. It is very common, occurring in about one in ten schoolchildren. The classical account of the features and management can be found in the late John Apley's excellent book *The Child With Abdominal Pains* (Apley, 1975). In most cases it is psychogenic, but before this diagnosis is made one needs to be satisfied that there is positive evidence of emotional disturbance and that demonstrable organic disease is absent. Apley was able to demonstrate organic disease in one child in 20, with renal tract abnormalities being the largest group.

In the majority the pain is located at the umbilicus and John Apley made the important observation that the further the site of the pain from the umbilicus, the more likely it is to be organic. Some attacks of pain are accompanied by nausea, pallor or vomiting and with a severe attack the child may be brought to hospital for assessment as to whether or not he has appendicitis. Appendicitis is common and these children are just as much at risk of having it as any other child. The history of previous bouts of abdominal pain does not exclude the diagnosis. A quarter of children admitted with appendicitis in the Southampton series were said to have experienced a similar episode of abdominal pain in the past. However, it is noteworthy that the incidence of appendicectomy is increased 16-fold in children with recurrent abdominal pain, and each episode has to be treated on its own merit.

When a thorough clinical evaluation and an MSU have revealed no sign of organic disease the family can be reassured. It needs to be explained that the pain is real and not imaginary, and is a common response to stress in children. It may be possible also to reduce some of the underlying environmental stress factors, which are often related to problems at school. Only a small minority are in need of specialist psychiatric treatment.

Long-term follow-up has shown a disappointing prognosis for the 'little belly-achers' whose problem was sufficiently severe to warrant referral to hospital. As adults, only a third are symptom-free, while a third continue to have abdominal pain and the remaining third have migraine or psychosomatic symptoms.

References

Apley, J. (1975), *The Child with Abdominal Pains*, Blackwell, Oxford.
Drake, D.P. (1980), *J. R. Soc. Med.*, **73,** 641.
Jackson, R.H. (1963), *Br. Med. J.*, **ii,** 277.
Meadow, R. (1979), *Arch. Dis. Child.*, **54,** 11, 822.

Further reading

Jones, P.G. (1976), *Clinical Paediatric Surgery*, Blackwell, Oxford.
Nixon, H.H. (1978), *Surgical Conditions in Paediatrics*, Butterworths, London.
Illingworth, R.S. (1979), *Common Symptoms of Disease in Children*, Blackwell, Oxford.

CHAPTER 7

Diabetic ketoacidosis and hypoglycaemia

There are approximately 30 000 diabetic children in Britain aged under 16 years. Each year there are about 1500 new cases and their age distribution is shown in Figure 1. Children with diabetes most often require emergency treatment when they develop ketoacidosis or if they become hypoglycaemic and this chapter describes these two situations.

Diabetic ketoacidosis

Before insulin became available, severe ketoacidosis was inevitably fatal. It remains a serious illness with a significant mortality, and requires obsessional care for a satisfactory outcome.

Diabetic ketoacidosis results from deficiency of insulin, the function of which is to conserve glucose in the body through its influence on a variety of tissues, particularly the liver, muscles and fat. The effects of lack of insulin are shown in Figure 2.

In the absence of insulin, glucose within cells becomes depleted and, despite high levels of extracellular glucose, the body responds as it would in starvation. Adipose tissue is broken down by lipolysis and large quantities of free fatty acids are produced. Simultaneously, muscle is catabolized and amino acids released into the circulation. In the liver these free fatty acids and amino acids are utilized in gluconeogenesis. The amino acids provide the carbon skeleton for

119

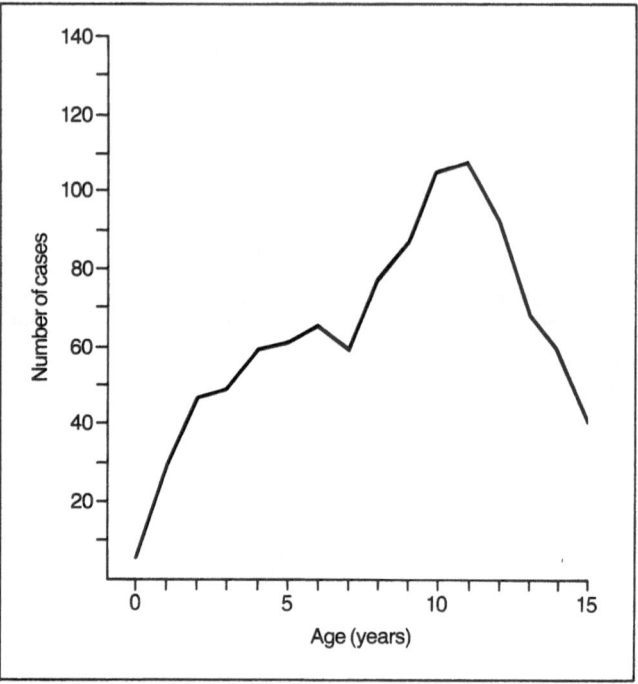

Figure 1 *Age distribution of new cases of diabetes in one year notified to the register of the British Diabetic Association. (Courtesy of the BDA)*

glucose, while the energy for its formation is produced by the break-down of the free fatty acids. Ketone bodies (3-hydroxybutyrate, aceto-acetate and acetone) are produced by these reactions and are released from the liver into the circulation. Glucose continues to be absorbed from food in the stomach. At the same time, the formation of glycogen in the liver is inhibited and glycogen stores are broken down to produce even more glucose. The lack of insulin also prevents the uptake of glucose by muscle and adipose tissue.

All these processes contribute to the rise in plasma glucose which exceeds the renal threshold and causes an osmotic diuresis, with loss of water and sodium. This fluid and electrolyte loss causes dehydration, which is further aggravated by vomiting and hyperventilation, and if severe may progress to shock.

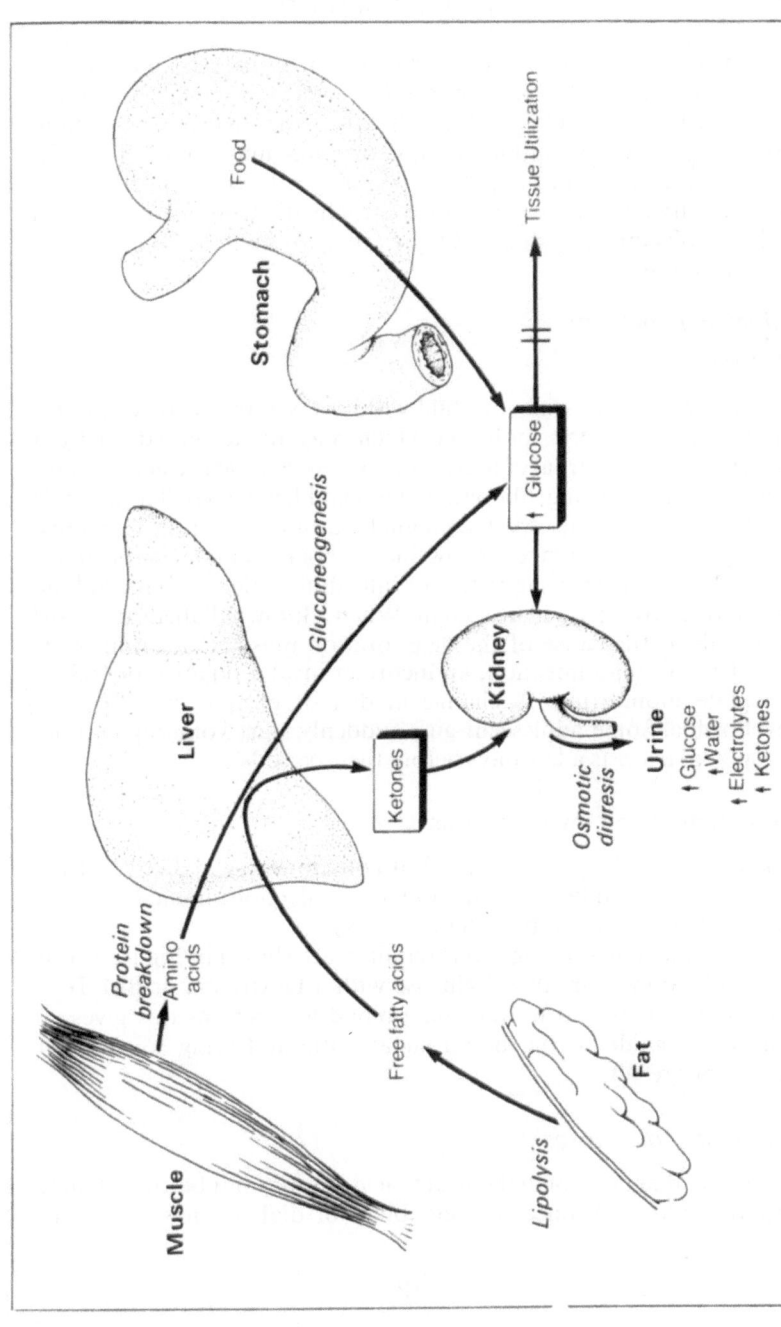

Figure 2 *Consequences of insulin deficiency*

A metabolic acidosis occurs, caused chiefly by the ketoacids, 3-hydroxybutyric and aceto-acetic acids, and exacerbated by the decrease in H^+ excretion which results from impaired renal function. Hyperventilation, vomiting and loss of potassium from cells result. Profound acidosis and hypokalaemia may adversely affect cardiac contractility and the patient will eventually die from a combination of hypovolaemia, hypoxia and myocardial malfunction unless treatment is initiated.

Initial management

History

A newly-presenting diabetic child will have symptoms reflecting his fluid loss, with thirst, polyuria which may be accompanied by a recurrence of nocturnal enuresis, and weight loss. More acute symptoms include vomiting, abdominal pain and headaches. The acidosis will produce characteristic Kussmaul breathing, and if the metabolic derangement is prolonged, drowsiness, shock and coma will supervene. Any symptoms suggestive of infection, which may precipitate the ketoacidosis, should be sought. When a known diabetic develops ketoacidosis the cause of the deterioration must be determined. It may be due to an infection, an incorrect insulin regimen or lack of adequate monitoring. A change in diet or exercise may also be responsible. Some adolescent girls suddenly start vomiting and develop ketoacidosis a few days before their periods.

Examination and investigations

The degree of dehydration, level of consciousness and state of the circulation should be assessed. Sources of infection should be sought and the patient should be weighed.

The immediate investigations required are shown in Figure 3. It is advisable to measure blood glucose with a Dextrostix or BM-Test-Glycemie '20-800' strip every time blood is taken, as this gives an immediate guide to the blood sugar without having to wait for laboratory results.

Differential diagnoses

The initial diagnosis of diabetic ketoacidosis may not be immediately apparent although once the possibility of diabetes has been con-

Blood glucose (Dextrostix and laboratory) and ketones

Urea, Na, K and bicarbonate, osmolality

Blood gases

Full blood count

Blood culture, MSU and chest radiograph

Lumbar puncture if indicated

ECG for T waves and ECG monitor

Body weight

Figure 3   *Immediate investigations required once ketoacidosis has been diagnosed*

sidered, and a urine sample obtained and tested, the diagnosis is usually straightforward and will be confirmed by the markedly elevated blood glucose. Other conditions which may occasionally cause confusion are pneumonia, salicylate overdose and acute abdominal pain.

Pneumonia

An abnormal pattern of breathing features in both diabetic ketoacidosis and pneumonia. The Kussmaul breathing of metabolic acidosis is characterized by an increased respiratory rate with deep respirations and no pauses between breaths, while in pneumonia, although the respiratory rate is also raised, the breaths are rapid and shallow. Of course, the two may coexist.

Salicylate overdose

Kussmaul breathing may also result from metabolic acidosis following salicylate overdose. These patients may also have glycosuria, though it is usually only a trace, and they may also be mildly hyperglycaemic. A positive Phenistix test of the urine will indicate the presence of salicylate, although a diabetic may have taken some aspirin. If there is difficulty distinguishing between the two conditions, a serum salicylate level can be estimated.

Acute abdomen

It is not always appreciated that diabetic ketoacidosis may be accompanied by severe abdominal pain. It can so exactly resemble an acute surgical emergency, with marked tenderness and guarding that the child may be admitted under the care of a surgeon. Marked dehydration and hyperventilation will usually help distinguish the diabetic from a true surgical condition, but occasionally an acute abdomen and diabetic ketoacidosis may occur together.

Principles of treatment

Treatment needs to be directed towards several features of the condition simultaneously. Although giving insulin is essential, the initial life-saving measure is fluid and electrolyte replacement. Water is required to correct the dehydration, sodium to expand the plasma volume and insulin to reverse the metabolic derangement. Without insulin the intracellular fluid becomes depleted of potassium, but once insulin has been given potassium will be transported into cells and will result in hypokalaemia unless preventive action is taken. The acidosis will gradually resolve but if it is very severe sodium bicarbonate can be given to prevent cardiac malfunction.

The management described below is for a child with profound ketoacidosis. Milder cases may not need such dramatic measures and each child must be assessed individually. Some newly presenting diabetics require subcutaneous insulin only, but the presence of moderately severe dehydration (more than 5%) is usually an indication for intravenous therapy.

Intravenous fluid

The first priority after the initial blood samples have been taken is to establish an intravenous infusion. This should be started immediately, aiming to give 10 to 20 ml/kg of 0.9% saline in the first hour.

If the patient is in shock, or peripheral circulatory collapse seems imminent, this should be replaced by 20 ml/kg of plasma. This initial resuscitation will allow time for organizing the biochemistry results and the insulin and calculating the subsequent fluid requirements.

The total fluid needed is the sum of the fluid deficit and the subsequent maintenance requirements (Figure 4). The fluid require-

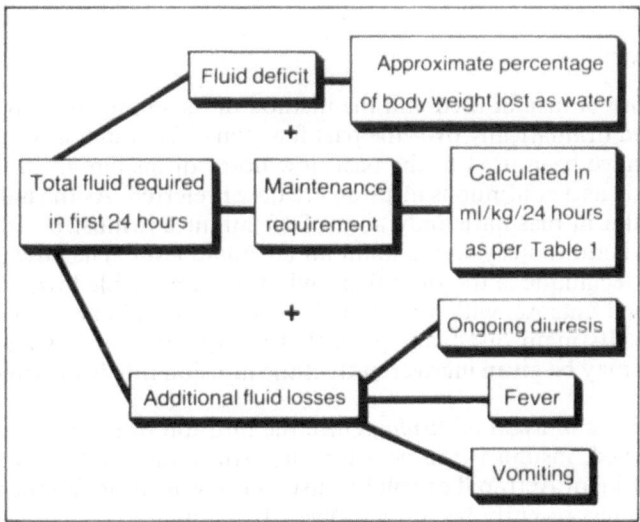

Figure 4   *Calculation of fluid replacement required. Half the total fluid required should be replaced in the first eight hours and the second half in the next 16 hours*

ment must be carefully calculated as it will vary according to the child's size. The degree of dehydration can be assessed clinically by estimating the approximate percentage of total body weight lost as water and a recent weight will be a useful guide. A child who has clinical signs of dehydration can be assumed to be 5% dehydrated and one who is hyperventing or has an impaired level of consciousness can be assumed to be at least 10% dehydrated (see Table 3 in Chapter 5).

A simple scheme is to calculate the total fluid requirement for the first 24 hours and give half of it in the first eight hours and the rest in the following 16 hours. In the first hour 10 to 20 ml/kg of 0.9%

125

saline is given, followed by 0.45% saline. This compromise will continue to expand the plasma volume without causing sodium overload, and is not so hypotonic as to cause a very rapid reduction of the serum osmolality. When the blood glucose falls below 14 mmol/l (250 mg%) the intravenous fluid should be changed to 4.2% dextrose/0.18% saline. Table 1 gives a guide to this scheme of fluid replacement and Figure 5 shows how it was used for an eight-year-old boy.

Insulin

The dose of insulin used and the method of its administration have changed dramatically over the past few years. Although large bolus doses have been used in the past, low doses of insulin given intravenously as a continuous infusion are now preferred. As the half-life of insulin in plasma is only about four minutes it must be administered continuously to maintain an adequate level. The advantage of this technique is the smoother and more predictable lowering of the blood glucose, with a lower risk of hypokalaemia and hypoglycaemia. Its main disadvantage is that a large dose of intravenous insulin may be given inadvertently if the infusion rate is incorrect.

Intravenous infusion of insulin. Once the infusion of saline has been established, insulin is the next priority. An initial loading dose of 0.1 unit/kg of Actrapid or soluble insulin is given, although the need for this has recently been questioned. It is followed by a constant insulin infusion of $0.1 \text{ unit kg}^{-1} \text{h}^{-1}$. The most satisfactory method of administration is with a syringe pump (Figure 6). If no syringe pump is available, an alternative method of giving a constant infusion is to use a paediatric giving set with an infusion pump and to add the insulin to the burette (Figure 7). Alternatively, hourly boluses of insulin of $0.1 \text{ unit kg}^{-1} \text{h}^{-1}$ can be given quite satisfactorily. The insulin should not be added directly to the main intravenous infusion as accurate control cannot be achieved. Nor should it be administered subcutaneously as its absorption will be unpredictable and erratic in the face of dehydration or shock. Another method is to give the insulin as hourly intramuscular injections, which works satisfactorily but has the disadvantage that the child is traumatized unnecessarily by repeated injections.

The aim is for the blood glucose to fall at approximately $4 \text{ mmol l}^{-1} \text{h}^{-1}$ $(75 \text{ mg } (100 \text{ ml})^{-1} \text{h}^{-1})$; a rate much faster than this

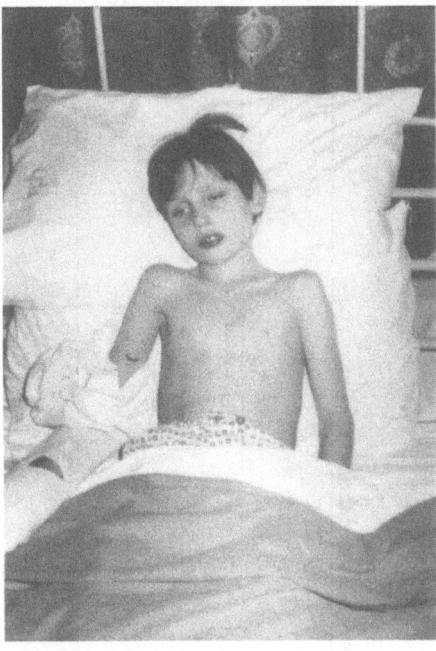

This eight-year-old boy was admitted severely dehydrated and acidotic. His condition had been precipitated by a chest infection. The method of calculating his fluid therapy was:

$$\text{Total fluid required in first 24 h} = \text{Deficit} + \text{Maintenance}$$
$$\text{Deficit} = 10\% \text{ of body weight (25 kg)}$$
$$= 2500 \text{ ml}$$
$$\text{Maintenance} = 1875 \text{ ml} (75 \text{ ml kg}^{-1} (24 \text{ h})^{-1} \text{ as per Table 1)}.$$
$$\therefore \text{Total fluid} = 2500 + 1875$$
$$= 4375 \text{ ml}$$

$$\text{In the first eight hours, half the total was given} = 2187 \text{ ml}$$

$$\text{In the first hour, 20 ml/kg of 0.9\% saline was given} = 500 \text{ ml}$$

In the next 7 hours (2187–500) ml = 1687 ml of 0.45% saline was given at 240 ml/h until the blood sugar fell below 12 mmol/l, when the infusion was changed to 4.2% dextrose/0.18% saline.

In the following 16 hours, the remaining half of the total fluid requirement was given = 2187 ml (135 ml/h) as 4.2% dextrose/0.18% saline

Figure 5   *Management of a child admitted with severe ketoacidosis*

Table 1   Guide to intravenous fluids in first 24 hours of severe ketoacidosis

Age (years)	Average weight (kg)	Deficit from 10% dehydration	Maintenance fluid total for 24 hours (ml/kg)	Volume of 0.9% saline in first saline (20 ml/kg)	Volume of 0.45% saline in next seven hours (ml/h)	4.2% dextrose/0.18% saline over next 16 hours (ml/h)
1	10	1000	1200 (120)	200	125	70
4	15	1500	1500 (100)	300	170	90
6	20	2000	1600 (80)	400	200	110
8	25	2500	1875 (75)	500	240	135
10	30	3000	1950 (65)	600	265	155
12	40	4000	2200 (55)	800	325	195

is undesirable. Rehydration alone in the first hour will usually result in a fall in blood glucose of 2 to 4 mmol/1 (34 to 75 mg/100 ml).

If there is no fall in blood glucose within two to four hours of starting this regimen, the rate of the insulin infusion should be doubled as there are occasionally patients who require a larger dose, particularly if they are severely acidotic. Although a 'low dose' regimen is recommended, one should not give too little insulin, as enough must be given to reverse the metabolic derangement.

Potassium

Profound ketoacidosis results in a marked deficit in total body potassium. This is greater in newly-diagnosed diabetics where the ketosis is of gradual onset than in known diabetics where it develops acutely. Potassium is lost in the urine, but plasma levels are maintained at the expense of intracellular potassium. The initial plasma potassium may be high and significant hyperkalaemia can be diagnosed on an ECG before any potassium is added to the infusion. For this reason potassium supplements should not be started until insulin has been given, but it is important not to delay replacement or severe hypokalaemia may result. It is not necessary to wait for a child to pass urine unless he is in shock, when ischaemic damage to the kidneys may occur. Underlying chronic renal impairment is extremely uncommon in diabetic children.

In general, 26 mmol KCl/1 (2 g/l) will prevent hypokalaemia, but this may have to be modified in the light of plasma potassium results. If the initial plasma potassium is above 6 mmol/l, wait until it falls below this level. Continuous ECG monitoring is advisable to detect arrhythmias and is mandatory in the exceptional instances when the concentration of KCl given is greater than 30 mmol/l. In severe cases of ketoacidosis oral potassium supplements (2 g KCl/day) may be needed for a week to overcome whole-body potassium depletion.

Bicarbonate

Use of sodium bicarbonate should be reserved for severe metabolic acidosis. In most cases, acidosis will resolve with rehydration, which improves tissue perfusion and reduces lactic acid production, and with insulin, which will stop any further production of ketoacids. However, very severe acidosis may adversely affect myocardial

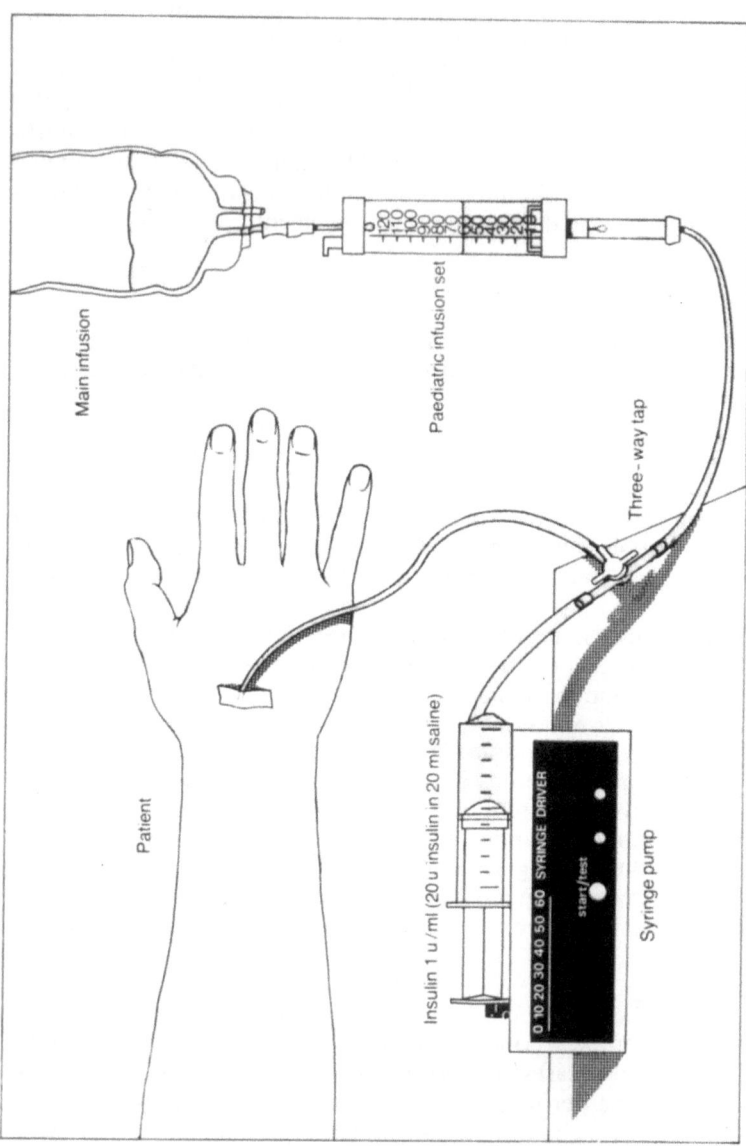

Figure 6 *Method of administering insulin intravenously with a syringe pump*

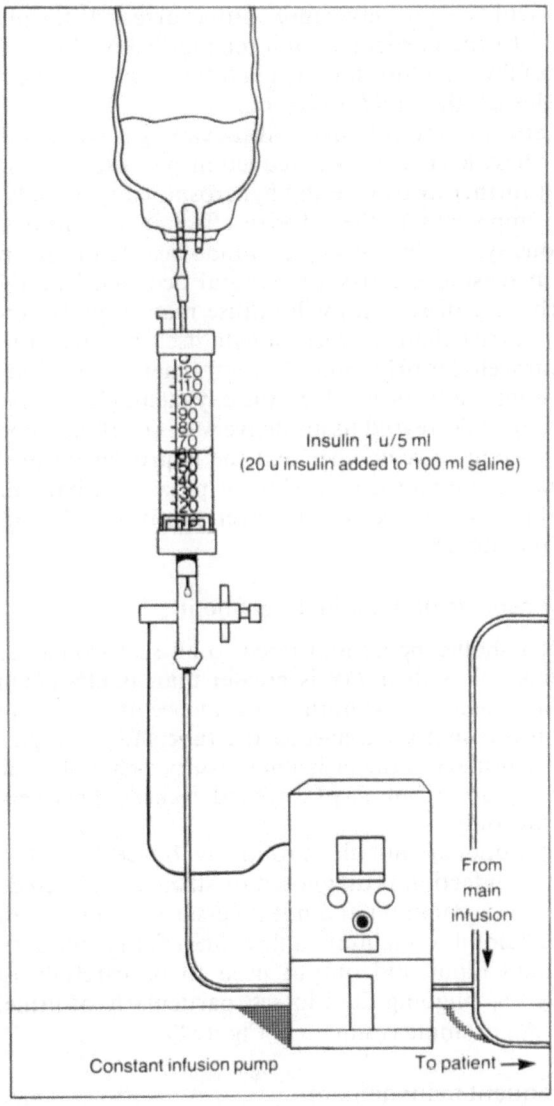

Figure 7   *Intravenous insulin infusion using a paediatric giving set*

contractility, and may cause cardiac arrest. If the plasma pH is less than 7.10 and particularly if it remains below this level after the first hour of fluid and insulin, then half the base deficit can be slowly corrected using the standard formula.

There are several major disadvantages in giving bicarbonate, which have led to a marked reduction in its use. As it is hyperosmolar, it will further aggravate the hyperosmolality already present. Even more important is the adverse effect it may have on the central nervous system by causing a paradoxical fall in the pH of the CSF and increasing the risk of cerebral oedema. The CO_2 into which bicarbonate dissociates will diffuse more rapidly across the blood-brain barrier than the bicarbonate itself and result in a decrease in the intracellular pH within the central nervous system. Furthermore, bicarbonate adversely affects the oxyhaemoglobin dissociation curve resulting in decreased tissue delivery of O_2. If bicarbonate is given, it is important to remember that the improvement in the plasma pH will be accompanied by a shift of potassium back into cells; additional potassium needs to be given intravenously and its level carefully monitored.

Other aspects of the initial treatment

Oxygen should be administered to all semi-comatose or comatose patients unless their Po_2 is greater than 10 kPa (75 mmHg). Where there is a history of vomiting or evidence of gastric dilatation, or the patient is comatose, a nasogastric tube should be passed and aspirated. A urinary catheter is unnecessary and undesirable if the child is passing urine, but may be needed in cases of severe shock to assess the urine output.

Antibiotics are not given routinely, but reserved for cases where a bacterial infection is diagnosed or strongly suspected. A high white cell count is common and not necessarily an indication of infection.

It is helpful to maintain a flow sheet for results and fluid balance. The fluid input and output need to be carefully and repeatedly checked as ongoing fluid losses, particularly of urine, may be very large. An example is shown in Figure 8.

Subsequent management

After the initial emergency treatment subsequent management must be planned according to each individual's response. Hypoglycaemia

Time from admission (h)	Fluid input				Fluid output				Laboratory results							Investigations
	Intravenous fluids										Na⁺		K⁺		Blood gases	
	0.9% Saline	0.45% Saline	4.2% Dextrose 0.18% Saline	Total	Urine	Other losses	Total	Blood glucose	Dextrostix		Bicarb-onate	Urea				
Arrival																Urea · electrolytes. blood glucose. blood gases. Dextrostix
1																
2																Urea · electrolytes. blood gas or bicarbonate. blood glucose · Dextrostix
3																
4																Dextrostix
5																
6																Urea · electrolytes, blood glucose,Dextrostix

Figure 8 Flow chart for fluid therapy and laboratory results

and hypokalaemia are the main problems which may occur early in treatment, and it is important to prevent these by close monitoring. Blood samples for glucose, electrolytes and bicarbonate or pH can be taken at two hours, six hours and thereafter depending on the patient's progress. More frequent checks on the blood glucose should be made with Dextrostix or BM-Test-Glycemie '20-800' in the first few hours.

If there is no steady response to initial treatment, a careful search for infection, particularly pneumonia or urinary tract infection, must be made. The occasional patient who suddenly deteriorates may have developed cerebral oedema

Blood glucose and electrolyte status is usually under reasonable control within 6 to 24 hours after admission. At this stage continuous insulin infusion can be changed to intermittent subcutaneous injection. Most children will require $0.05-2$ units $kg^{-1}(24 h)^{-1}$ of Actrapid. If desired a sliding scale, using urine or blood glucose levels, can be used to assess the dose of Actrapid to be given every six to eight hours (Table 2). Sips of oral fluid can usually be introduced

Table 2   Sliding scale for urine or blood glucose levels

Urine glucose (g/100 ml)	Blood glucose		Dose of subcutaneous Actrapid to be given six-hourly (Units/kg)
	(mmol/l)	(mg/100 ml)	
5	>20	>360	0.5
2–3	16–20	290–360	0.4
1	13–16	235–290	0.3
0.5	10–13	180–235	0.2
0–Trace	<10	<180	0.1

For urine, use the 'two-drop' method: 2 drops urine + 10 drops of water + a Clinitest (Ames) tablet

within 6 to 24 hours and then food also when these are well tolerated. As control is achieved the Actrapid can be given before meals three to four times a day and eventually a once- or twice-daily regimen can be introduced.

134

Hypoglycaemia

Diabetic children and their parents should be able to recognize the symptoms and signs of hypoglycaemia. These vary between children, but tend to be consistent for an individual.

Early hypoglycaemia may be accompanied by a change in personality, with temper tantrums, tearfulness or laughing. Other children complain of dizziness, headaches, sudden hunger or they may become pale or flushed or temporarily develop a squint. In more severe instances coma or convulsions occur. Nocturnal hypoglycaemia may be associated with nightmares, abnormal behaviour or convulsions. It is usually advisable for a newly-diagnosed diabetic to experience mild hypoglycaemia so that he will be familiar with his own reaction to it. This can be done most satisfactorily before discharge from hospital by giving the usual dose of insulin in the morning but delaying breakfast for a few hours. The sympathomimetic reaction to hypoglycaemia and to anxiety or stress is similar and distinguishing between them can be very difficult, particularly in the young child. Indeed, there may be many false alarms. In such instances home monitoring of blood glucose with a BM-Test-Glycemie '20-800' strip or a Dextrostix reflectance meter can be of great assistance.

Hypoglycaemia represents a failure in diabetic control. The causes of hypoglycaemia are shown in Table 3. In all cases it is most

Table 3   Causes of hypoglycaemia in diabetes

Excessive insulin	—reduced requirement, e.g. 'honeymoon' period
	—alteration in the regime
	—overdose, accidental or deliberate
Reduced glucose intake	—meals missed or delayed
	—vomiting or anorexia in infection
Increased utilization of glucose	—exercise

important that the cause is ascertained so that appropriate therapy can be instituted for the acute episode and action taken to prevent its recurrence. The cause may result from a breakdown in the understanding of the child or his parents of the inter-relationship between the dose of insulin, diet, exercise and home monitoring of urine or blood glucose. There are three periods when children are particularly vulnerable to hypoglycaemia, these being the period after diagnosis, that following a change in insulin from a standard to a monocomponent form and during infection.

Excessive insulin can easily be given in the weeks following the initial diagnosis of diabetes, the 'honeymoon' period, when insulin requirements often fall dramatically. Similarly, patients who are changed from a standard to a monocomponent preparation will require on average about a third less than their previous dose, but this is variable and a recent series showed that many patients become hypoglycaemic (Griffin *et al.*, 1979). During intercurrent infection, insulin requirements are increased and higher doses of insulin are usually given accordingly. If the child vomits or becomes anorexic this increased dose may prove excessive and result in hypoglycaemia.

Management

Early hypoglycaemia

When a child or his parents notice the symptoms of hypoglycaemia, preventive action should be taken by eating glucose tablets or lumps of sugar, or else by having a glucose-containing drink. All diabetics

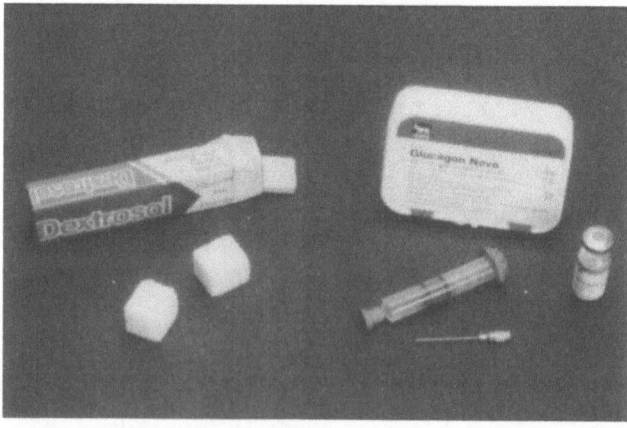

Figure 9   *Early hypoglycaemia can be controlled by taking sugar lumps or glucose tablets; intramuscular glucagon can be given by parents if the child is unconscious*

and the parents of young diabetic children should carry glucose tablets or sugar lumps with them wherever they go (Figure 9). Adults who are left in charge of diabetic children, particularly school teachers, should be aware of the problems and know how to deal with them. (The explanatory leaflet for teachers—*The Diabetic At School*—issued by the British Diabetic Association, 10 Queen Anne St, London W1, is useful.) A snack or meal should be eaten after a hypoglycaemic episode.

Severe hypoglycaemia

The diabetic child who suddenly becomes unconscious and unable to take any sugar orally requires emergency treatment. Convulsions are common in children with severe hypoglycaemia. An intramuscular injection of 1 mg of glucagon will usually restore consciousness sufficiently for the child to take oral glucose. Parents should keep an ampoule of glucagon at home in the refrigerator, and be able to give the injection (Figure 9). If the child is not at home or no glucagon is available medical assistance should be urgently obtained. On arrival

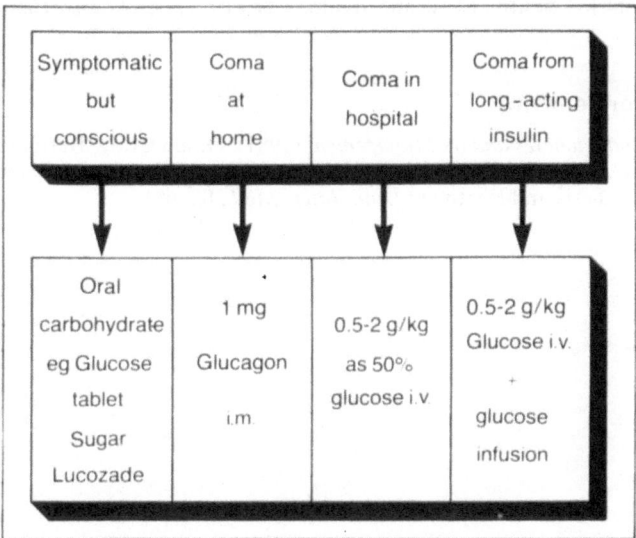

Symptomatic but conscious	Coma at home	Coma in hospital	Coma from long-acting insulin
Oral carbohydrate eg Glucose tablet Sugar Lucozade	1 mg Glucagon i.m.	0.5-2 g/kg as 50% glucose i.v	0.5-2 g/kg Glucose i.v. + glucose infusion

Figure 10   Summary of the management of hypoglycaemia

137

at the accident and emergency department the immediate therapy is to give 50% dextrose intravenously, to a maximum of 2 g/kg or 4 ml/kg. The dextrose should be diluted with an equal volume of water, otherwise it is so viscous that it is difficult to inject and is highly sclerotic. If there is any delay in establishing an intravenous infusion, glucagon should be given. A Dextrostix and blood glucose should be carried out and in most cases will be less than 2.5 mmol/l (45 mg/100 ml). An intravenous infusion may need to be continued if the hypoglycaemia has resulted from an excess of long acting insulin. A summary of the management of hypoglycaemia is shown in Figure 10.

Although many texts have tables contrasting the difference between hypo- and hyperglycaemic coma, the known diabetic child who suddenly becomes unconscious from hypoglycaemia presents a totally different clinical picture to the child who has slowly become dehydrated and acidotic from ketoacidosis. Distinguishing between the two rarely presents any difficulty.

References

Griffin, N.K., Smith, M.A. and Baum, J.D. (1979), *Arch. Dis. Child.*, **54,** 123.

Further reading

Childhood Diabetes and its Management (1981), Oman Craig, Butterworths.
Kreisberg, R.A. (1978), Diabetic ketoacidosis: new concepts and trends in pathogenesis and treatment. *Ann. Inter. Med.*, **88,** 681.

CHAPTER 8

The febrile child

Fever is one of the commonest presenting features of illness in children. Self-limiting viral infections are usually the cause but it is always important to distinguish these from more serious infections which will need treatment and it is these which will be emphasized in this chapter. Of prime importance is the child's age as the most likely cause, the mode of presentation, the physical signs and the appropriate therapy will all be influenced by this.

Symptomatic treatment for the fever itself should be given both for the comfort of the child and to reduce the likelihood of febrile convulsions. The child should be kept cool by removing excess clothing and by tepid sponging but if the water used is too cold vasoconstriction and shivering are induced which can increase the core temperature. Oral paracetamol should be given regularly rather than waiting for a recurrence of fever. Paracetamol and aspirin are equally effective as antipyretics but aspirin is used less widely because of the higher incidence of side-effects.

Age less than two months

Very young babies are immunologically immature and are susceptible to an enormously wide range of organisms. Serious illnesses present with minimal, nonspecific symptoms and signs and it is advisable for all babies in this age group who are febrile to be admitted to hospital. A fever is usually present in an infected baby but not always and there may be an unstable temperature or even hypothermia. Other symptoms and signs of infection are listed in Table 1. Reluctance to feed is an early symptom and vomiting and diarrhoea, lethargy or irritability and cyanotic or apnoeic episodes may also signify the onset of an infection. In meningitis the specific signs of a bulging anterior fontanelle, convulsions or lying in an opisthotonic posture are usually only late features.

Table 1   Symptoms and signs of infection in infants less than two months old

Symptoms	Signs
Generally unwell	Fever, hypothermia or unstable body
Reluctance to feed	temperature
Vomiting	Hypotonia
Diarrhoea	Jaundice
Lethargy	Convulsions
Irritability	Splenomegaly
Cyanotic or apnoeic attacks	Purpura
	Hypoglycaemia

Investigation

The vagueness of the symptoms means that any baby of this age in whom there is any suspicion of infection will need thorough investigation. The basic tests are listed in Table 2. A raised neutrophil count, especially an increase in the proportion of immature neutrophils, may accompany an infection but a neutropenia is even more significant and is seen with severe infections. Blood cultures must always be taken as septicaemia is particularly common in this age group because infections are not well localized. Suprapubic aspiration of urine is the surest way of diagnosing or excluding a urinary

Table 2   Investigations which may be needed in an ill baby

Full blood count
Blood culture, blood glucose, urea and electrolytes
Chest radiograph
Suprapubic aspiration of urine
Lumbar puncture
Blood gas
Swabs from skin, ear and umbilicus

tract infection. It is indicated if the baby is seriously ill and the cause unknown. Lumbar puncture is performed even in the absence of specific neurological signs and the CSF should be gram stained and examined under the microscope, as well as cultured, whether white cells are present or not. The normal range of CSF results in the newborn is wider than in older children (Table 3) and this results in a greater overlap between normal and abnormal results. When microscopy is negative or the child has been on antibiotics counter-current immunoelectrophoresis may be helpful.

Table 3   CSF in the normal term neonate

	Mean	Range
WBC (cells/mm³)	8	0–32
Protein (g/l)	0.9	0.2–1.7
Ratio of CSF glucose to blood glucose	0.8	0.45–2.5

Pathogens

The immaturity of the host defences at this age—especially in preterm infants—is reflected by the wide range of pathogens encountered and includes organisms normally considered to be of low virulence or contaminants. Gram-negative organisms particularly *E. coli* and *Pseudomonas aeruginosa* are the commonest causes of serious infections but these have been overtaken by group B β-haemolytic streptococcal infections in some centres. Group B streptococci are found in maternal vaginal flora at about 15% of deliveries and approximately half these babies are found to carry it on their skin. However, only 0.1% of all babies become infected. Group B streptococcal disease tends to take two separate forms characterized by early- and late-onset disease. The early form presents usually within the first 48 hours after birth, with respiratory distress and septicaemia, whereas the late form presents at two to four weeks of age, most commonly as meningitis but also as osteomyelitis or pneumonia. Whereas the early form tends to follow a rapidly progressive course, the late-onset disease may be more insidious. Both have a high mortality.

Treatment

A baby of this age with an untreated bacterial infection may well deteriorate clinically or die within a matter of hours. This makes it necessary to start antibiotics promptly, before culture results are available. Broad spectrum antibiotics are required, with penicillin or ampicillin in high doses, to cover group B streptococci, other Gram-positive organisms and *Listeria monocytogenes*. These are combined with an antibiotic which is effective against the Gram-negative organisms. Gentamicin is usually used and levels need to be monitored to ensure that drug levels are adequate but not excessive. Antibiotics are given systemically as oral absorption is particularly unreliable at this age.

In meningitis the morbidity and mortality of Gram-negative infections remains high because of the difficulty of eradicating the organism from the ventricles (Figure 1). This may not be possible with gentamicin even if it is given intrathecally or into the ventricles (Siegel and McCraken, 1981). Chloramphenicol tends to be used in this situation in England (Drugs and Therapeutic Bulletin, 1981) as it

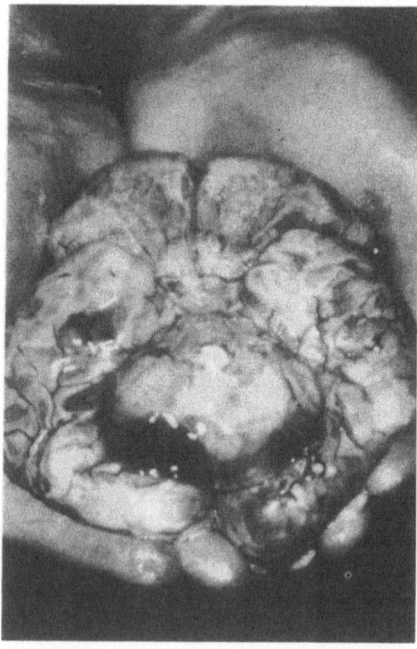

Figure 1 *Postmortem appearance following* E. coli *meningitis in spite of vigorous antibiotic therapy*

crosses into the CSF well but the dose needs to be modified in preterm infants and the drug levels closely monitored to avoid the 'grey baby' syndrome.

Age greater than two months

To consider all children over two months old in one group is clearly an over-simplification. As children grow older their immune system gradually matures and their susceptibility to different pathogens changes. The signs and symptoms at presentation are also determined by the child's age and progress from the vague ill-defined changes of the sick neonate to the specific and localizing features of the older child. The threshold for admission to hospital and for performing a comprehensive septic screen including a lumbar puncture is thus much lower the younger the child.

Most children with an acute febrile illness have an upper respiratory tract infection or one of the common infectious diseases. A watch must be kept for the child with coryzal symptoms, sore eyes and Koplik's spots on the buccal mucosa to avoid admitting a child with measles to a general ward. When children have returned from tropical countries malaria and typhoid should be remembered. A description of these and the many other causes of fever in a child will not be attempted, but instead only a few which need prompt recognition and treatment will be described.

Otitis media

The main difficulty in the diagnosis of acute otitis media lies in obtaining a good view of the eardrum and in interpreting what is seen. Redness of the tympanic membrane alone can be seen in any child who is febrile or crying. Valuable additional criteria are the loss of landmarks and light reflex and bulging of the tympanic membrane. A pneumatic auroscope attachment should be available and impaired mobility of the eardrum can then be observed.

From the neonatal period onwards, the pneumococcus is the commonest bacterial organism responsible. Next most common in children less than six years old is *Haemophilus influenzae*, while in the older child it is the group A β-haemolytic streptococcus. In many cases no organism can be identified. Suitable antibiotics are co-trimoxazole (Septrin, Bactrim) or amoxycillin (Amoxil) in the

143

young child and penicillin in the older. Decongestants may help drainage through the eustachian tubes. Hearing deficit is common following otitis media and follow up should be arranged to ensure that there has been complete resolution.

Periorbital cellulitis

With periorbital cellulitis there is fever, malaise and unilateral periorbital swelling with discoloration of the skin. The cellulitis usually develops as a complication of acute sinusitis or as an extension of facial cellulitis which may follow injury to the skin (Figure 2). The organisms involved are usually staphylococci, streptococci or, in children under two years of age, *Haemophilus influenzae*. Prompt treatment should be instituted, with intravenous antibiotics to prevent the infection spreading to involve the orbit. In true orbital cellu-

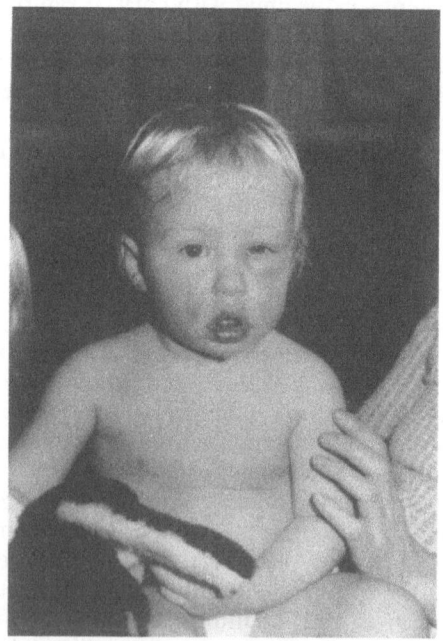

Figure 2   *Periorbital cellulitis from a spreading facial cellulitis*

litis the eyelids are red and oedematous, and there is orbital pain and proptosis. Ophthalmoplegia may develop.

Infective endocarditis

This occurs predominantly in children with congenital heart disease, particularly with tetralogy of Fallot, ventricular septal defect and valvar aortic stenosis. The first blood culture reveals the pathogen in most cases, but the yield can be increased by culturing several specimens of blood in the first 24 hours or in a shorter period if the child is very ill.

Osteomyelitis

With osteomyelitis the infected bone is painful and held immobile. There is exquisitely painful point tenderness which may be elicited by tapping anywhere along the bone. The affected part may be swollen and erythematous. An adjacent joint may also be swollen with a sympathetic effusion. Early signs are unwillingness to move the affected bone or to weight bear. The limbs and spine of all children with an unexplained fever must be carefully examined and palpated for evidence of local swelling and tenderness. This is especially true for infants where the illness may be more insidious with less constitutional disturbance and the signs less obvious.

A neutrophil leukocytosis and raised ESR are often seen but are non specific. The organism can often be identified on blood culture. Radiographs taken early in the illness show only soft tissue swelling, and it is only after about 5 days in an infant or 10 days in older children that subperiosteal new bone formation and bone destruction are seen. Radio-isotope bone scans will be abnormal at presentation and are particularly helpful when the clinical signs are equivocal, especially in babies or if the child has already been on antibiotics. A needle aspiration of the bone may be performed to isolate the organism but the current trend is to reserve this or other surgical procedures for patients who have failed to respond to antibiotics. A diagnostic biopsy may be necessary in some cases to differentiate infection from a bone tumour particularly Ewing sarcoma or a primary bone lymphoma.

Prompt and effective antibiotic therapy is crucial to avoid bone necrosis, sinus formation and limb deformity. In children over 2 months, *Staphylococcus aureus* is by far the commonest organism, with *Haemophilus influenzae* and *Streptococcus pyogenes* isolated much less frequently. Salmonella osteomyelitis is seen especially in children with sickle cell disease. High dose antibiotics are given intravenously for one to two weeks followed by oral antibiotics. A suitable choice of antibiotics would be flucloxacillin and fusidic acid.

Septic arthritis

In septic arthritis the joint is hot, swollen and acutely tender, movement is severely restricted and painful. Children may be febrile and toxic, but as with osteomyelitis the infant may present with general malaise, and be noted subsequently to be holding a joint in a fixed position and resisting movement. This is seen especially in septic arthritis of the hip, which is first noticed when the leg is kept flexed and adducted, and there is gradual swelling around the adductor region of the hip and genitalia. Osteomyelitis in a bone may result in a sterile sympathetic effusion of an adjacent joint but in the hip joint there may be direct spread of infection as the femoral metaphysis lies within the joint capsule.

In all cases the joint should be aspirated and the fluid examined by microscopy and culture. Blood should also be cultured. A radiograph taken early on may show only capsular distortion, but a hot spot can be demonstrated on a bone scan.

Antibiotics must be started promptly to avoid serious damage to the joint. This is especially important with the hip where severe destruction can develop very rapidly and early drainage of the joint by an orthopaedic surgeon will be needed. The choice of antibiotic will depend on the organism identified. *Staphylococcus aureus* is the commonest and can be treated with intravenous flucloxacillin and fusidic acid. *Haemophilus influenzae* is not uncommon in children between 2 months and 4 years and can be treated with chloramphenicol. More than one joint may be affected and the infection may spread to other sites, particularly the meninges. The joint is rested in its position of function with plaster or traction and as the infection subsides physiotherapy is introduced to improve muscle function. Even after antibiotics have been started the joint must be kept free of pus as it is very lytic to cartilage. Repeated aspiration of the joint may be required, but if the pus is loculated or there is not a prompt response to antibiotic therapy, surgical exploration will be necessary.

Urinary tract infections

The older child may complain of dysuria or frequency. Other clinical features are abdominal pain, either acute or recurrent, loin pain or a fever. Dysuria also occurs in the acute urethral syndrome, from balantitis or acute vulvitis. Symptoms are much less specific in the young child. Acute symptoms are fever, febrile convulsions, vomiting or diarrhoea, or the presentation may be more chronic with poor feeding or failure to thrive. A sample of urine needs to be taken for microscopy and culture from every sick child. The management is discussed in more detail on page 202.

Meningococcal septicaemia

Meningococcal septicaemia is usually a severe febrile illness of rapid onset and progression and is not always associated with meningitis. It is usually identified by the accompanying purpuric rash (Figure 3)

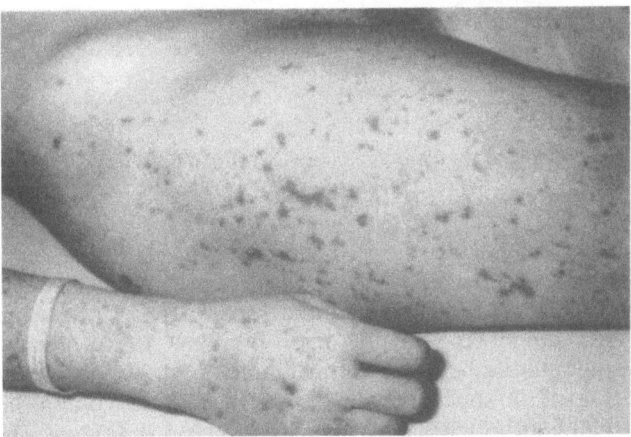

Figure 3 *Characteristic purpuric rash of meningococcal septicaemia*

which varies from a few small and scattered petechiae to the classic extensive coalescing purpura with areas of necrosis. In the most fulminant form, adrenal haemorrhage (Waterhouse-Friderichsen syndrome) and circulatory collapse occur and disseminated intravascular coagulation may also be present (Figure 4). The main problem

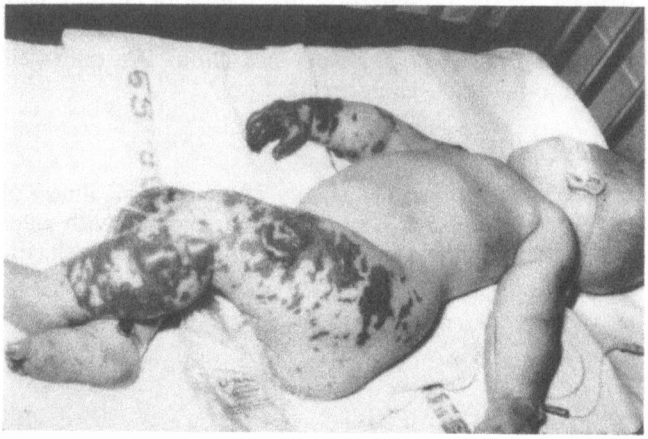

Figure 4 *Fulminant meningococcal septicaemia. The head is retracted from meningitis*

is delay in recognizing the rash and instituting treatment. In an analysis of a number of fatal cases of meningococcal infection in Britain, the petechiae or confluent haemorrhagic rash were seen but the correct diagnosis was not made (Oakley, 1979). Penicillin in high dosage should be started immediately and given intravenously. If the child is in shock expansion of the plasma volume may be required and, although the plasma cortisol level is not low, pharmacological doses of steroids are often advocated. (See Septic shock, p. 192.)

Bacterial meningitis

Bacterial meningitis is predominantly a disease of childhood, with over half of all cases occurring in children aged less than four years.

It has been estimated that the risk for a child living in London of developing an acute meningococcal infection is 1 in 1000 and for *Haemophilus influenzae* meningitis, 1 in 1500 (Goldacre, 1976).

The more characteristic symptoms and signs appear only in older children, with fever, vomiting and severe headaches often accompanied by photophobia. In more advanced cases the child may be delirious or comatose, have convulsions and lie with the head retracted. Children less than two years old may have nonspecific signs and, as in the neonate, a bulging fontanelle occurs late, but drowsiness, lethargy or irritability should arouse suspicion. It is uncommon for a child with a convulsion from meningitis to be thought to have had only a febrile convulsion but in children below two years old it is safest for a lumbar puncture to always be performed after a first febrile convulsion. The same applies to older children unless one is confident that they do not have meningitis. Examination of a child with suspected meningitis may reveal clues to its origin, such as

	Excess polymorphs	Excess lymphocytes
Glucose ↓ Protein ↑ ↑	Bacterial meningitis Tuberculosis Mumps meningoencephalitis	
Glucose normal Protein ↑ or normal	Early viral meningitis Viral meningitis Polio Tuberculosis Brain abscess	

Figure 5 *CSF findings in meningitis*

149

middle ear disease, basal skull fractures or a dermal sinus. Any purpura will suggest meningococcal sepsis. A child who has already been given antibiotics may have less florid symptoms and the threshold of suspicion must be high.

The presence of genuine neck stiffness is the most helpful sign. As most children will resist forcible flexion of the neck and neck stiffness may be incorrectly diagnosed, it is more helpful to ask the child to watch a toy or torch and test the range of neck movement indirectly. An alternative method is to ask them to kiss their knee. Kernig's sign is usually positive: the hip and knee are initially flexed and on extension of the lower leg there is pain in the hamstrings and the back. However, Brudzinski's sign, where forcible flexion of the neck produces flexion of the knees is both unpleasant and unnecessary.

True neck stiffness must be differentiated from meningism which is not uncommon in children with a high temperature and tonsillitis, pneumonia—particularly of the upper lobes—and tender cervical lymphadenopathy.

The CSF changes caused by agents other than bacteria are shown in Figure 5. In bacterial infection the causative organism can usually be seen on gram stain of the CSF, otherwise it may be identified on culture of the CSF or blood. Three organisms are responsible for the vast majority of cases: *Neisseria meningitidis*, *Streptococcus pneumoniae* and, in children less than six years old, *Haemophilus influenzae* (Table 4). An organism may not be grown in a child who has been partially treated with antibiotics although the pleocytosis will still be evident.

Table 4   Causes of meningitis at different ages

Less than two months
   Gram-negative organisms, especially *E. Coli*
   Group B β-haemolytic streptococcus
   Listeria monocytogenes

Two months to six years
   Haemophilus influenzae
   Neisseria meningitidis
   Streptococcus pneumoniae

Children over six years
   Neisseria meningitidis
   Streptococcus pneumoniae

Management

If the CSF is turbid, intravenous antibiotics should be started immediately. There is no generally accepted antibiotic regimen but one which covers pneumococcus, meningococcus and *Haemophilus influenzae* must be chosen. A combination of penicillin ($120\,\text{mg}\,\text{kg}^{-1}$ $(24\,\text{h})^{-1}$)—which is the drug of choice for pneumococci and meningococci—together with chloramphenicol (50 to $100\,\text{mg}\,\text{kg}^{-1}\,(24\,\text{h})^{-1}$) against *Haemophilus influenzae* is often used. Ampicillin in very high doses ($400\,\text{mg}\,\text{kg}^{-1}\,(24\,\text{h})^{-1}$) was a satisfactory alternative until recently, but strains of *H. influenzae* resistant to ampicillin are being increasingly isolated. In North America a combination of high dose ampicillin and chloramphenicol is widely used. The drugs can be adjusted once the culture results are known.

If the child is shocked initial resuscitation will be required. Once the plasma volume has been restored fluids should be restricted to one-third to two-thirds of normal maintenance levels, both to counteract inappropriate antidiuretic hormone secretion and to minimize cerebral oedema.

Convulsions occur in about a quarter of the cases and will need to be treated. Subdural effusions are most common with *Haemophilus influenzae* but they also occur in pneumococcal infections. It may be possible to demonstrate their presence by transillumination, ultrasound or CT scan but they are not usually tapped unless there is a deterioration in the child's condition. Hydrocephalus may also develop acutely. On recovery any hearing deficits especially after infection by *Haemophilus influenzae* need to be identified. Long term sequelae include ataxia, deafness and mental retardation ranging from poor school performance to severe handicap.

Prophylaxis

In meningococcal meningitis, the attack rate for intimate household contacts in increased one-thousandfold. Sulphonamides will effectively eliminate the nasopharyngeal carrier state, but 18% of organisms are now sulphonamide-resistant. Several studies have shown that rifampicin will eliminate nasopharyngeal carriage of the meningococcus in over 90% of patients. As prophylaxis for intimate household contacts should be given immediately, before antibiotic sensitivity is known, rifampicin (Rifadin) is often recommended

(Wilson, 1981). It should not be given to pregnant women and is awkward if soft contact lenses are worn, as conjunctival secretions become orange in colour. Any close contact who becomes unwell should be promptly evaluated.

With *Haemophilus influenzae* meningitis, there is also a marked increased incidence of secondary attacks in household contacts below four years of age. Rifampicin has been given to families when there is a susceptible child at home (rifampicin 600 mg b.d. for adults, $20 \, \text{mg kg}^{-1} (24 \, \text{h})^{-1}$ for children 1 to 12 years old, $10 \, \text{mg kg}^{-1}$ $(24 \, \text{h})^{-1}$ if less than one year old, for four days).

Children with an increased risk of infection

A group of children with an increased risk of infection are encountered in any paediatric department. Primary immunodeficiency is uncommon but much more common is secondary immunosuppression induced by drugs, especially steroids and the chemotherapeutic agents used to treat malignant disease. These children are also vulnerable to infections by unusual organisms including fungi and *Pneumocystis carinii*. During courses of chemotherapy they are likely to have periods of neutropenia. If the absolute neutrophil count falls below $0.5 \times 10^9/\text{l}$ ($500/\text{mm}^3$) the risk of bacterial infection increases dramatically and a febrile child with this white cell count should be admitted to hospital, have cultures and screening tests performed, and be treated with broad-spectrum antibiotics (for example azlocillin and gentamicin (Genticin)). These children are also at serious risk throughout their therapy from varicella and measles which can cause overwhelming and fatal disease. If they are known to be susceptible they should try to avoid contact with infected children. If they do come into contact with varicella they should be treated with zoster immune globulin within the first 48 hours. Should they become infected (Figure 6) a course of acyclovir (Zovirax) may be considered. This is an acyclic nucleoside which has been found to have a high level of antiviral activity in vitro against viruses of the herpes group, and is currently being assessed in clinical trials.

Children without a spleen have a markedly increased risk of contracting pneumococcal disease including septicaemia, peritonitis, and meningitis, or infections caused by other encapsulated organisms, particularly *H. influenzae* and *Salmonella*. This may occur following surgical removal of the spleen or as a result of functional asplenism

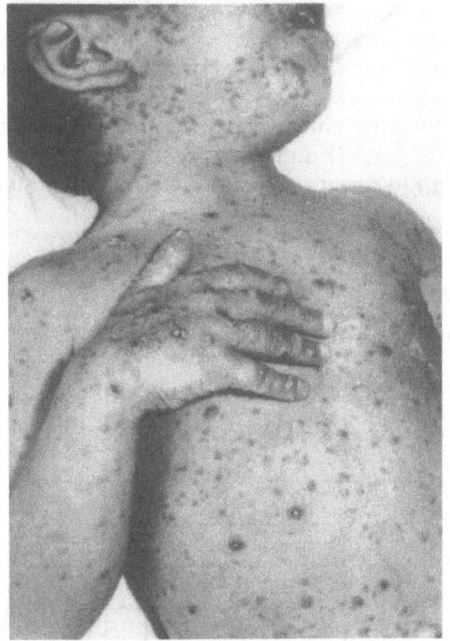

Figure 6 *Haemorrhagic varicella in an immunodeficient child*

as in sickle cell disease. Younger children are at greater risk. This risk is sufficient for many paediatricians to recommend continuous prophylactic penicillin for these patients. A pneumococcal vaccine (Pneumovax) is now available and may provide immunity in children aged over two years against 14 of the most common North American strains. Children with nephrotic syndrome are also particularly vulnerable to pneumococcal disease while they have proteinuria and may be given prophylactic penicillin.

Prolonged fever

In a large series from Boston of children with unexplained fever persisting for more than two weeks, an infective cause was the final diagnosis in half the cases (Pizzo *et al.*, 1975). The largest number were viral, but bacterial causes included urinary tract infections,

153

infective endocarditis, osteomyelitis, typhoid and tuberculosis. The other important causes are connective tissue disorders, malignancy, regional ileitis, and mucocutaneous lymph node syndrome—a recent addition to the list.

In systemic juvenile chronic arthritis (Still's disease), there is a high, intermittent fever (Figure 7). The most common age of presentation is less than five years, when there is an equal incidence in boys

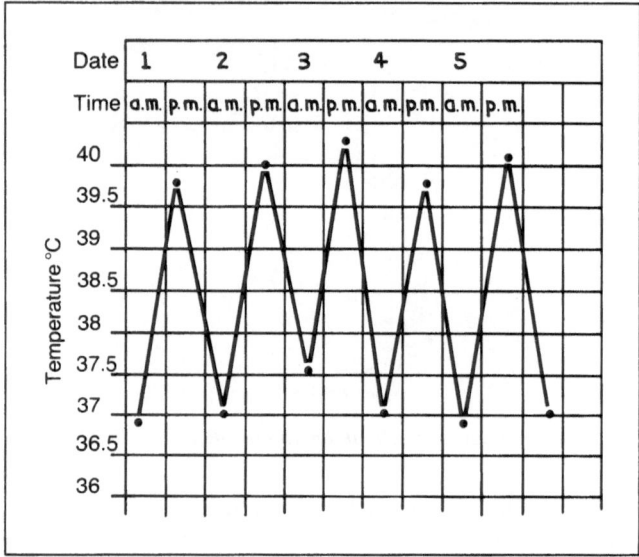

Figure 7 *Characteristic pattern of fever in systemic juvenile chronic arthritis*

and girls. The child is toxic and unwell, and almost all patients have a characteristic maculopapular rash, which is most pronounced at the height of the fever. Other features include generalized lymphadenopathy, splenomegaly, hepatomegaly and pericarditis. Ultimately, most will develop arthritis but this may not be present at first. There is a marked polymorphonucleocytosis, the ESR is extremely high and a mild anaemia usually occurs. The most difficult differential diagnosis used to be rheumatic fever, but this is now rarely seen in the indigenous population. An initial haemoglobin less than 10 g would make one very suspicious of malignant disease (Ansell, 1980).

Leukaemia and non-Hodgkin's lymphomas may present with an unexplained fever or with many of the same features as systemic juvenile chronic arthritis.

Regional ileitis (Crohn's disease) may present with high fevers and is often accompanied by anorexia, weight loss and abdominal pain, although this latter symptom may not be prominent in a young child.

Mucocutaneous lymph node syndrome (Kawasaki's disease) causes diagnostic difficulties in the early stages in a child who is clearly very unwell. Several thousand cases have been described in Japan (Kawasaki *et al.*, 1974) and since then many cases have been identified in North America and Europe. The main clinical features are listed in Table 5. The peak age range is 12 to 18 months and most

Table 5   Diagnostic features of mucocutaneous lymph node syndrome

Fever
Spiking, lasting five days or more

Eyes
Bilateral conjunctivitis

Mouth
Lips dry, cracked and red
Erythematous oropharyngeal mucosa

Hands and feet
Reddening of palms and soles on day three to five with desquamation by the second or third week

Trunk
Macular erythematous rash

Cervical lymph nodes
Enlarged

are younger than five years old. There is a high, spiking fever which may continue for two to three weeks, and the child is toxic. Other initial features are conjunctivitis, dry, cracked and red lips, deeply erythematous oral mucosa, and cervical lymphadenopathy (Figure 8). The most distinctive feature is the pronounced reddening of the palms and soles, with indurative oedema of the hands and feet which develops after three to five days of the illness, followed at two to three weeks by desquamation of the tips of the fingers and toes (Figure 9). The disease carries a 1-2% mortality from cardiac

155

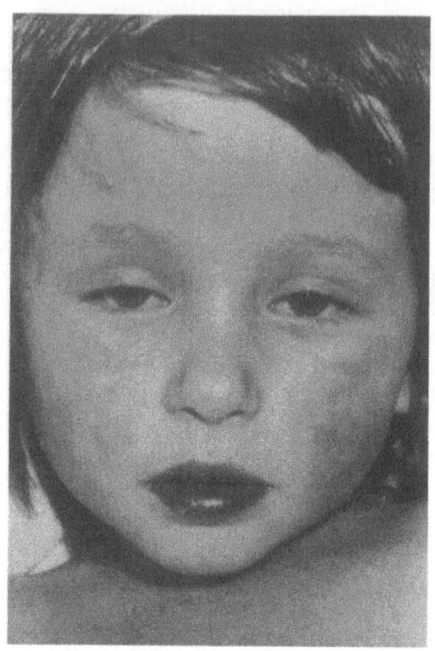

Figure 8   *Facial appearance in mucocutaneous lymph node syndrome showing red cracked lips and rash*

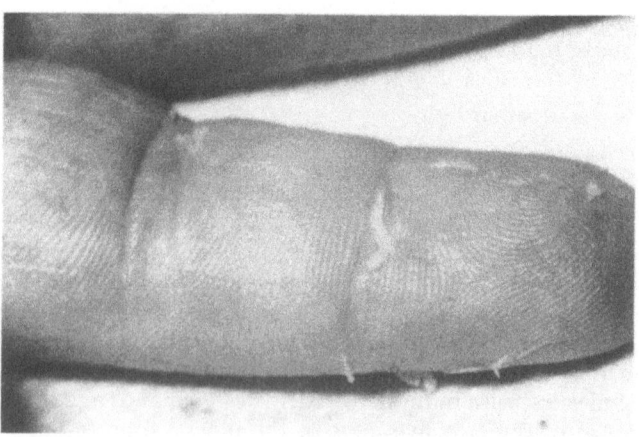

Figure 9   *Desquamation of the tips of the fingers in mucocutaneous lymph node syndrome*

involvement. The pathological findings are indistinguishable from infantile polyarteritis and the disease may result in aneurysms and thromboses in the coronary arteries. Death occurs as a result of myocardial infarction or rarely from cardiac arrhythmias or rupture of an aneurysm.

References

Ansell, B.M. (1980), *Rheumatic Disorders in Childhood*, Butterworths, London.

Goldacre, M.J. (1976), *Lancet*, **i,** 28.

Kawasaki, T., Kosaki, F., Okawa, S., Shigematusi, I. and Yanagawa, H. (1974), *Paediatrics*, **54,** 271.

Oakley, J.R. and Stanton, A.N. (1979), *Br. Med. J.*, **ii,** 468.

Pizzo, P.A., Lovejoy, F.H. and Smith, D.H. (1975), *Paediatrics,* **55,** 468.

Further reading

Antibacterial chemotherapy in the newborn, *Drugs and Therapeutics Bulletin 1981*, **19,** 4.

McCracken, G.H. and Nelson, J.D. (1977), *Antimicrobial Therapy for the Newborn*, Grune and Stratton, New York.

Siegel, J and McCracken, G.H. (1981), Sepsis neonatorum, *N. Engl. J. Med.*, **304,** 642.

Wilson, H.D. (1981), Prophylaxis in bacterial meningitis, *Arch. Dis. Child.*, **56,** 817.

CHAPTER 9

Convulsions

A child's threshold to have a convulsion and the clinical pattern it takes depend on the brain's stage of maturation. Between one and six months of age, the threshold is high and convulsions are uncommon. When they do occur, they are often partial, fragmented and disorganized, or if generalized take the form of infantile spasms. In contrast, in children between six months and five years old, the threshold to convulse is particularly low, with a fever often acting as the trigger. Other seizure disorders, which may be generalized, that is, tonic-clonic, petit mal or myoclonic, or else partial seizures, are also seen at this age.

Infantile spasms

The age of onset of infantile spasms is between three and nine months. In 1841 Dr West described the onset of these spasms in his own son in a letter to *The Lancet*. He noted that they were sudden, bilateral spasms with flexion of the neck, trunk and hips, with the arms initially abducted and then flexed. He also described the subsequent intellectual regression. Very occasionally the spasms are extensor. The convulsions are often in clusters, terminating in a cry or scream, and occur particularly when the child is dropping off to sleep or awakening. There is frequently marked developmental deterioration, particularly in psychosocial development and this may be the reason for the parents seeking medical advice. The EEG is characteristic and shows a totally disorganized pattern with almost continuous spikes and discharges, referred to as hypsarrhythmia (Figure 1).

Infantile spasms are an age-related reaction to a wide variety of

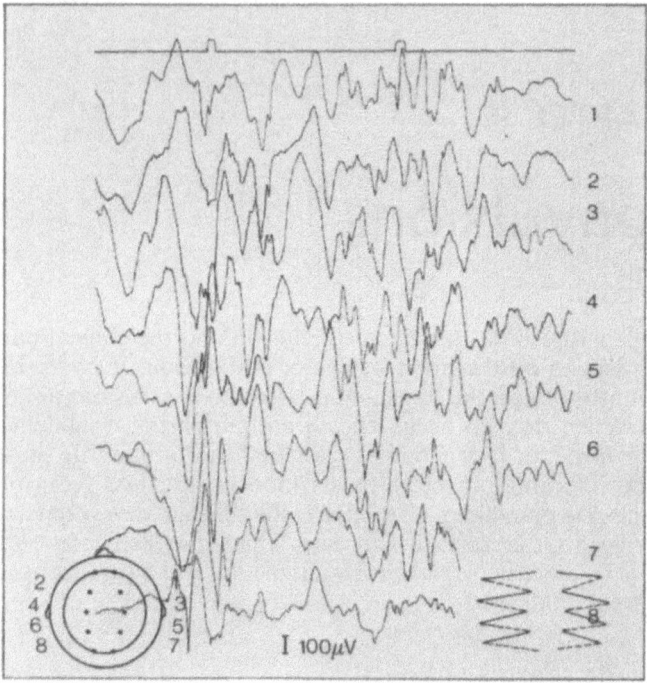

Figure 1 *Hypsarrhythmia, the characteristic EEG in infants with infantile spasms. There is total disorganization with almost continuous spike and polyspike discharges*

insults. Two-thirds of these infants have a generalized neurological disorder (the symptomatic group) and in many, developmental delay or abnormalities will already have been identified. There are many causes, but two important ones are severe perinatal insults and tuberose sclerosis (Figure 2).

The remaining third of these infants are in the cryptogenic group, whose development has been normal and where there is no apparent

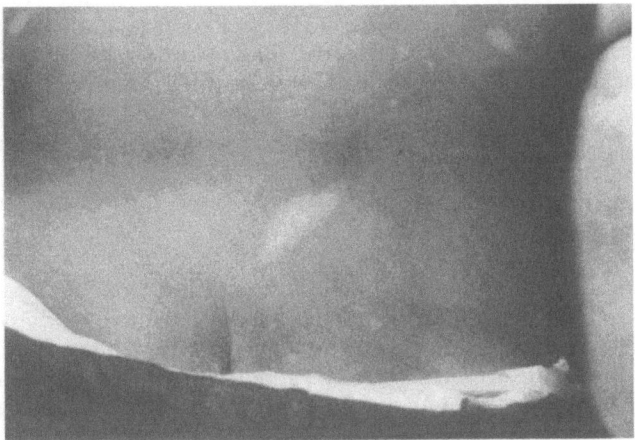

Figure 2 *White patches of depigmentation which may first be detected with ultraviolet light, may be the initial clue to the diagnosis of tuberose sclerosis*

underlying cause. Very occasionally, infantile spasms may start shortly after pertussis immunization, but the relationship between the two is uncertain.

Therapy with steroids or benzodiazepines has been used (Table 1). Steroids given to infants in the cryptogenic group are often followed by the disappearance of the infantile spasms and improvement in the EEG, and up to half may develop normally. The earlier treatment is started, the better the outlook. Various combinations of both ACTH and prednisolone in high dosage have been used. When a neurological disorder is present, although drug therapy will often initially suppress the seizures and improve the EEG, it does not alter the

Table 1   Initial therapy of infantile spasms in infants

Cryptogenic group
ACTH 40 units/24 h for one to two weeks, followed by:

Prednisolone $2 \, mg \, kg^{-1} (24 \, h)^{-1}$ for four to six weeks, then tail off over a similar period

Symptomatic group
Clonazepam 0.5 to 1 mg/24 h (initially 0.25 mg/24 h), or
Nitrazepam 2.5 to 7.5 mg/24 h

161

progression of mental retardation. The benzodiazepines nitrazepam (Mogadon) or clonazepam (Rivotril) tend to be used for these infants as they do not have the serious side-effects of high-dose steroids. Their use may be limited by drowsiness or increased bronchial secretions. In many infants, the infantile spasms relapse or may be followed by other types of convulsions.

Febrile convulsions

Febrile convulsions are common, affecting 3 to 4% of children. They are a terrifying experience for parents and indeed many are convinced that their child is about to die. Not only are they one of the most common reasons for children to be admitted to hospital acutely but many aspects of their management continue to be controversial and so they will be described in some detail.

Certain children are particularly susceptible to convulse with an acute febrile illness. This is highly age-dependent and occurs between six months and five years old, with a peak incidence between 9 and 20 months. It is thought that the rapid rise in temperature is more important than the ultimate height of the fever in precipitating the convulsion. Viral infections particularly of the upper respiratory tract are most often the cause. Other vulnerable periods are the prodromal phase of roseola infantum or measles and during shigella infections. By definition a child admitted with a convulsion associated with a fever cannot be considered to have a febrile convulsion unless there is no evidence of intracranial infection or any underlying neurological cause for the convulsion.

The typical history is that the child has been unwell and febrile, and then suddenly convulses. The convulsions usually last only a minute or two. The eyes roll upwards and generalized tonic-clonic movements occur. Unconsciousness with cyanosis or pallor is present but frothing at the mouth and biting the tongue are not features at this age.

Usually the convulsion has stopped by the time the child reaches hospital, but if not, the airway should be cleared and the child placed in a semiprone position and given oxygen. The convulsion should be stopped with anticonvulsant drugs if it lasts longer than five minutes. The fever must also be controlled by removing all the child's clothes, apart from a nappy or pants, and by tepid sponging. Regular antipyretics, usually paracetamol or else aspirin should be given.

The source of fever is often the throat or ears, but in particular meningitis should be excluded—although unusual, it may present with what initially appears to be a febrile convulsion. It is advisable for all children under two years of age to have a lumbar puncture following a convulsion associated with a fever, as meningitis cannot be confidently excluded clinically at this age. Lumbar puncture is also required in older children unless one is certain that they do not have meningitis. It may be difficult to make a reliable clinical assessment if the child is seen very soon after the fit and has not yet fully recovered. Although other investigations are rarely abnormal, a Dextrostix and blood glucose should be performed, and will in any case be required as part of the evaluation of the CSF. If no cause for the fever can be found, an MSU is essential, and a full blood count, blood culture and throat swab may be helpful.

Parents will need a careful and sympathetic explanation about febrile convulsions. They should also be advised on what to do when their child has other febrile illnesses in the future. Contrary to many parents' inclinations, these children should be kept cool with few clothes and regular antipyretics to try to prevent a rapid temperature rise. If a convulsion does occur they should ensure the child's airway is clear but not force anything into the mouth, lie the child semiprone with a pillow under the bottom and obtain urgent medical help if the convulsion has not stopped within five minutes. Giving the parents a pamphlet containing this information or writing it down for them is helpful.

Prognosis

In the past, febrile convulsions were regarded as benign, but more recently this view has been challenged and it is now accepted that severe febrile convulsions can result in epilepsy and subsequent neurological handicap. Prolonged febrile convulsions have been incriminated in the production of macroscopic damage to the hippocampal region, resulting in mesial temporal sclerosis, which is associated with temporal lobe epilepsy. While it is generally agreed that children who have had febrile convulsions are at increased risk of becoming epileptic, there is disagreement concerning the magnitude of the risk. In the Collaborative Perinatal Project in the USA, the progress of 54 000 children was followed, and 1706 of them had febrile convulsions (Nelson and Ellenberg, 1976). For the vast majority the prognosis was excellent. Risk factors for the development of afebrile seizures, both isolated and recurrent, were found to include the presence of abnormal developmental status prior to the convulsion, complex seizures, or family history of afebrile seizures (Table 2). Epilepsy by the age of seven years was found in 0.5% of

Table 2   Risk factors for the development of epilepsy

Presence of pre-existing abnormal neurological development
A complex febrile seizure:
Longer than 15 minutes or
Focal or
Followed by transient or persistent neurological abnormalities
Family history of non-febrile seizures in a parent or sibling

children who had never had a febrile convulsion, compared with 2% of those who had. The incidence of epilepsy is dramatically increased to 10% if two or more risk factors were present (Figure 3). In addition, febrile seizures were associated with an increased risk of intellectual deficit only among children with pre-existing neurological or developmental abnormality, and in those who developed subsequent afebrile seizures. Other studies have suggested that the major difference between benign febrile convulsions and those which are antecedents of epilepsy is in severity, as determined by length, frequency, age of onset, any previous brain injury and possibly the sex of the child (with young girls at higher risk) (Lennox-Buchtal, 1973).

Prophylaxis

There continue to be many different opinions about which children should receive prophylaxis and the form it should take. A third of children who have a febrile convulsion will have another, and 10% will have multiple convulsions. The younger the child at the time of the initial convulsion, particularly in girls, the higher the risk of recurrence. A child less than a year old has a 50% chance of a recurrence, and 30% experience more than one recurrence.

Measures to prevent further convulsions include keeping the child cool and giving regular antipyretics with any subsequent febrile illness, but convulsions occur in spite of these measures and in a third of cases there is no prior warning that the child is unwell.

CONVULSIONS

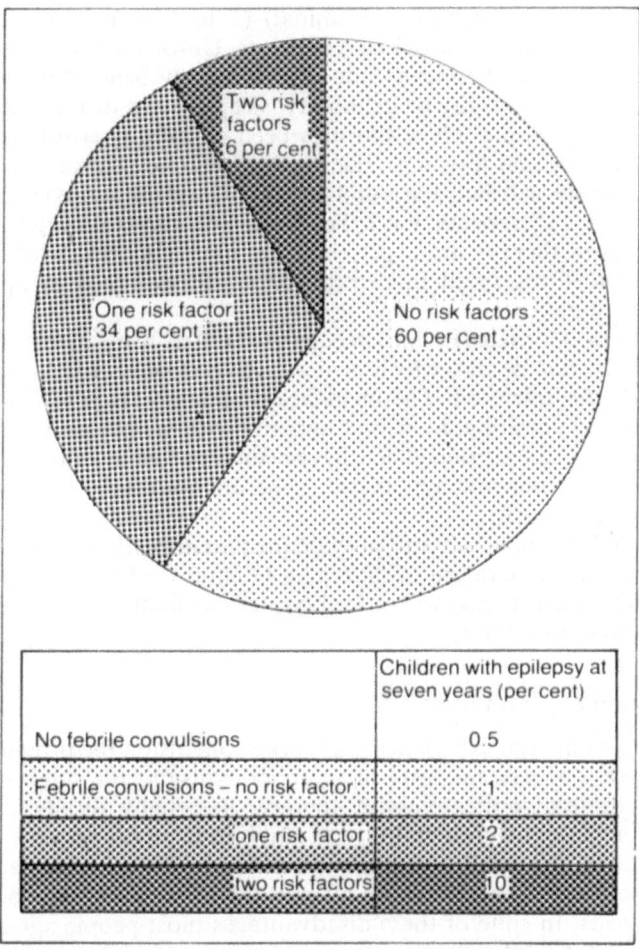

	Children with epilepsy at seven years (per cent)
No febrile convulsions	0.5
Febrile convulsions – no risk factor	1
one risk factor	2
two risk factors	10

Figure 3   *The incidence of epilepsy following febrile convulsions at seven years of age, and the influence of the risk factors listed in Table 2. (Data from the Collaborative Perinatal Project, Nelson & Ellenberg, 1976)*

Regular phenobarbitone (Luminal) (4 to 6 mg/kg once a day) significantly reduces the risk of recurrence. Unfortunately, up to 40% of children have significant side-effects, mainly behaviour disturbance with hyperactivity or irritability, sleep pattern disturbance and negative behaviour. There has also been concern over interference with memory and learning. The phenobarbitone needs to be given continuously on a daily basis and the serum level monitored to ensure an adequate therapeutic level. Transient side-effects during the first few days of therapy are experienced by most children, while long-term side-effects result in therapy being discontinued in up to a quarter of patients.

Sodium valproate (Epilim) may be used (20 to 30 mg kg^{-1} (24 h)$^{-1}$ in two divided doses), which is as effective as phenobarbitone and much better tolerated. The incidence of side-effects is low, mainly nausea and vomiting, increased appetite with weight gain and alopecia. Rare, serious side-effects have been reported including thrombocytopenia, marrow hypoplasia, hyperammonaemia, hepatic failure and pancreatitis.

A different approach is to provide the parents with a supply of the intravenous preparation of diazepam (Valium), which they can administer rectally (5 mg) with a 1 ml syringe (without a needle) as soon as a convulsion starts.

Selection of prophylaxis

For most children experiencing a febrile convulsion the prognosis is excellent. The vast majority of severe convulsions are single events and long-term anticonvulsant therapy has many disadvantages. These include the undesirability of children taking long-term medication, the side-effects, compliance, which is often unsatisfactory, and the necessity and expense of repeated medical supervision and blood tests. In spite of these disadvantages most people agree that there is a group of children with an increased probability of developing long-term sequelae who should receive prophylaxis, but considerable debate continues over which children constitute this high-risk group.

In the USA the National Institute of Health consensus statement recommends that prophylaxis be considered if any of the risk factors listed in Table 2 are present (NIH Consensus Statement, *British Medical Journal*, 1980). This would mean that a third of all children with febrile convulsions would receive prophylaxis. It is also recommended that prophylaxis should be carefully considered in children with recurrent convulsions or infants less than 12 months old. Prophylaxis is usually continued for at least two years, or one year after the last convulsion, whichever is the longer.

Conditions which may cause confusion

The diagnosis of a convulsion relies primarily on a detailed clinical history of the fit and the events surrounding it. Other important information is the family history and details from the perinatal period and the child's developmental progress. Other conditions may mimic a convulsion. In small babies, infantile spasms may be confused with colic, and there is often considerable delay before the diagnosis is made. In infants, febrile convulsions may not be easy to differentiate from rigors, or from the shivering which may accompany a high fever.

Breath-holding attacks are frightening and parents will usually seek urgent medical attention. The onset is usually between 6 and 18 months, and there are two forms, cyanotic and pallid. The cyanotic attacks are easier to recognize—the child suddenly starts to cry vigorously, but then stops breathing in expiration. Cyanosis follows after a few seconds, with transient loss of consciousness and floppiness. This may be accompanied by a few clonic twitches. Rapid recovery follows. The most characteristic feature is that there is always a precipitating cause, either a physical or a psychological injury. There is no significant relationship with subsequent epilepsy or mental retardation, and the attacks become less frequent after the age of three years. No medication is indicated.

'White' breath-holding attacks are much less common. They are triggered by relatively trivial stimuli, usually unexpected minor bumps to the head or sudden fright, after which the child goes very pale and loses consciousness. It is thought that they arise from vagal stimulation causing a prolonged period of asystole.

Status epilepticus

A severe continuous seizure or repeated fits with incomplete recovery of consciousness constitute status epilepticus. Young children are at much greater risk of sustaining brain damage in status epilepticus than adults, and may do so after a shorter period. After 30 minutes of a generalized tonic-clonic convulsion, the child is already in danger of sustaining permanent brain damage. Continuous fits for longer than 10 minutes should be terminated as a matter of urgency.

The commonest cause of a prolonged seizure in a young child is a prolonged convulsion associated with a fever. Children with epilepsy are particularly prone to convulse following changes in anticonvulsant therapy, and those with the Sturge–Weber syndrome or tuberose sclerosis may present with intractable fits. Intracranial infections are an important cause, and need to be considered in all children who have a convulsion.

Management

The child should be placed semiprone and oxygen given. An adequate airway must be maintained, by gently extending the neck and elevating the jaw. Blood should be taken for a Dextrostix and blood glucose to exclude hypoglycaemia, and for estimation of anticonvulsant drug levels if the child is already receiving therapy, as this will be helpful when reassessing the child's drug regime. Drugs will need to be given to control the seizure (Table 3). Diazepam (Valium) is the drug of choice, given slowly and intravenously; the response is usually very rapid. It may cause respiratory depression, especially if a barbiturate has previously been administered, but this is usually transient and will respond to mask and bag ventilation. Diazepam has a short half-life, and if fits recur, the bolus can be repeated after 20 minutes. Clonazepam (Rivotril) has been advocated as being superior to diazepam, but it may produce copious bronchial secretions and is not widely available.

The commonest difficulty is in establishing a reliable intravenous infusion in a convulsing child, particularly a chubby one. Diazepam is poorly absorbed if given intramuscularly but has been used rectally (5 mg), with good results. Paraldehyde remains a useful alternative, either when there is delay in establishing an intravenous infusion, or if the fits are resistant to an initial dose of diazepam. It needs to be given by deep intramuscular injection into the lateral side of the thigh to avoid the sciatic nerve. It may cause sterile abscesses, and its powerful smell is unpleasant, but other side-effects are very rare. Traditionally it is drawn up in a glass syringe, though it can safely be used in most plastic syringes, as long as it is given promptly.

Table 3   Antiepileptic drugs used in grand mal status epilepticus

Drug	Route	Dose	Side-effects
Diazepam	i.v.	0.3 mg/kg (or 1 mg/y of age + 1 mg) Maximum single dose 10 mg	Sedation Respiratory depression, particularly after phenobarbitone Thrombophlebitis
Paraldehyde	i.m.	1 ml/y up to 5 ml, or 0.1 to 0.15 ml/kg	Sterile abscesses
	p.r.	0.3 ml/kg	Mix with equal volume of mineral oil
Phenytoin	i.v.	15 to 20 mg/kg over 20 minutes	Hypotension Rarely cardiac dysrhythmias
Phenobarbitone	i.v.	5 to 10 mg/kg	Sedation Respiratory depression Hypotension

Both phenytoin (Epanutin) and phenobarbitone (Luminal), intravenously, are widely used in North America, but are usually regarded as second-line drugs in England. Phenytoin has the advantage of being less sedative and so does not obscure neurological signs. It must be given slowly over 20 minutes, and a syringe pump can conveniently be used for this. Hypotension is an uncommon side-effect, and cardiac arrhythmias are rare in the absence of pre-existing cardiac disease. It must be given with caution if the patient is already taking the drug. Phenobarbitone may also be used, but is slower to act, causes sedation and may lead to depression of respiration. Chlormethiazole (Heminevrin) has also been used with good effect. It is very easy to lose valuable time switching from one drug to another, and over-dosage with these hypnotic drugs can be dangerous. As has already been stressed it is the duration of status epilepticus prior to effective control that is critical in preventing death and residual neurological damage. If the seizure is proving refractory to adequate doses of two different drugs, then it is usually better to call for an experienced anaesthetist's help and give sodium thiopentone (Intraval sodium) to stop the convulsion. A continuous infusion may subsequently be required. Long-acting muscle paralysis is best avoided.

Following a very prolonged seizure, supportive management in an intensive care unit will be required and a long-acting anticonvulsant given if only short-acting drugs have been used to control the fit.

References

Lennox-Buchtal, M.A. (1973), *Electroenceph. Clin. Neurophysiol.*, Suppl. 32.
Nelson, K.B. and Ellenberg, J.H. (1976), *N. Engl. J. Med.*, **295,** 1029.
NIH Consensus Statement on Febrile Seizures (1980), *Br. Med. J.*, **281,** 277.
West. W.J. (1841), *Lancet*, **1,** 724.

Further reading

Addy, D.P. (1981), Prophylaxis and febrile convulsions, *Arch. Dis. Child.*, **56,** 2, 81.
Bower, B. (1978), The treatment of epilepsy in children, *Br. J. Hosp. Med.*, **19,** 1, 8.
Brown, J.K. and Sills, J.A. (1977), Status epilepticus, *J. Mat. Child Health*, **2,** 10.
O'Donohoe, N.V. (1979), *Epilepsies of Childhood*, Butterworths, London.

CHAPTER 10

Coma

The first priority in the management of a comatose child is to secure an airway and provide respiratory support if necessary. If the child is in shock, this must be reversed if possible (Chapter 11).

Thereafter, the cause of coma will need to be established and important causes are listed in Table 1. Excluding trauma, the main causes in children are intracranial infection and prolonged convulsions. Less common are Reye's syndrome, metabolic encephalopathies and drug ingestion.

Infections

Of the intracranial infections meningitis is the most frequently encountered and must be excluded in every child in coma unless the cause is known. In most cases the child will have a fever and neck stiffness. The management of bacterial meningitis caused by the most common pathogens, the meningococcus, *H. influenzae* and the pneumococcus is described on page 148. Tuberculous meningitis usually has an insidious onset with a tendency to affect the base of the skull resulting in cranial nerve palsies, but it may present as an acute encephalopathy with raised intracranial pressure. It is always associated with infection elsewhere in the body, usually in the lungs, and over 80% have an abnormal chest radiograph.

Cerebral abscess is a rare condition for which there is usually a predisposing cause such as a penetrating head injury, meningitis or

Table 1   Important causes of coma

CNS causes
Intracranial infections
    Meningitis
    Encephalitis
    Brain abscess
Fits and postictal states
Postanoxic encephalopathy
Head trauma
    Severe concussion
    Extradural or subdural haematomas
Cerebrovascular abnormalities
    Haemorrhage, thrombosis, emboli, infarct
    Hypertensive encephalopathy
Tumours

Systemic causes
Drugs and toxins
    Overdose: tricyclic antidepressants, salicylates,
    barbiturates, iron, alcohol, etc.
    Lead
Fluid and electrolyte abnormalities
Metabolic encephalopathies
    Hypoglycaemia and diabetic ketoacidosis
    Hepatic failure
    Renal failure
    Inherited metabolic disorders
Shock and overwhelming sepsis
Reye's syndrome

congenital heart disease, especially right to left shunts. It may also follow otitis media either from direct extension of a chronically infected ear, or from sinusitis or mastoiditis. There is a wide spectrum of clinical features, ranging from raised intracranial pressure to meningitis or focal neurological signs. The diagnosis can usually be made with a CT scan (Figure 1) and an urgent neurosurgical opinion must be sought. Therapeutic measures to reduce the cerebral oedema surrounding the abscess should be taken with mannitol and dexamethasone.

Encephalitis produces disturbed consciousness and fever, and

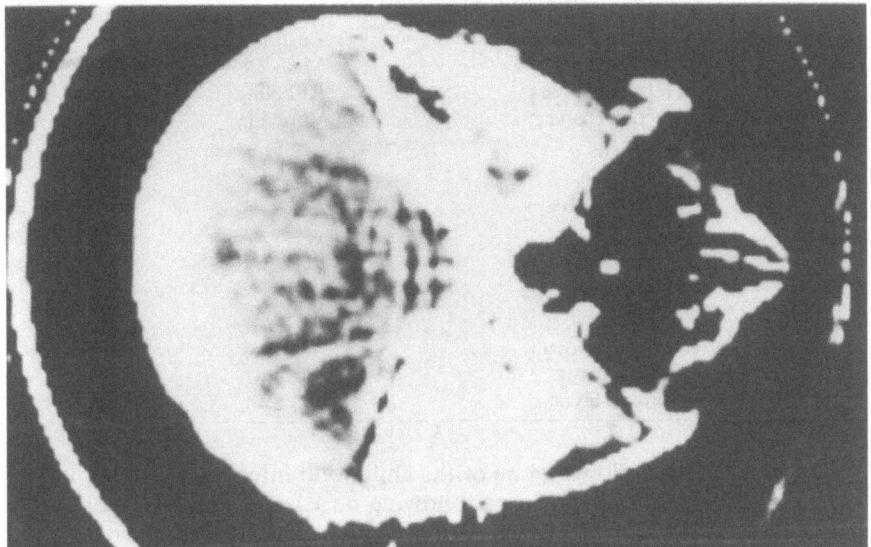

Figure 1 CT scan showing a cerebellar abscess in a child with a cholesteatoma

there may be convulsions and focal neurological signs. The majority
of cases are viral (Table 2). Herpes simplex encephalitis is the most
common sporadic severe encephalitis in which a virus is identified,
but it is rare. Only 10 to 15% of cases are associated with herpetic
gingivostomatitis or skin lesions. Focal convulsions and neurological
signs suggesting a temporal lobe lesion are frequent. The mortality is
extremely high, and there are often severe neurological sequelae in
survivors. The cerebrospinal fluid may initially be normal, but later
shows a lymphocytosis. EEG and CT scan may help in distinguishing
encephalitis from a cerebral abscess or a tumour, and show temporal
lobe abnormalities. Prompt identification is important as antiviral
therapy with adenosine arabinoside may reduce mortality if given
early (Whitley *et al.*, 1977). A new antiherpetic agent, acyclovir, is
currently under clinical trial and the preliminary reports of its
efficacy and very low toxicity are encouraging. A definitive diagnosis can only be made on brain biopsy, though therapy may be
begun using only clinical criteria and the results of the EEG and CT
scan.

Table 2   Causes of viral encephalitis

Infections	*Postinfectious*
Herpes virus	Measles
Herpes simplex	Rubella
Herpes zoster	Varicella
Enterovirus	
Coxsackie	
Poliomyelitis	
Echo	
Myxovirus	
Mumps	
Rabies	
Arthropod-borne	
Yellow fever	
Dengue fever	

Encephalitis following one of the childhood infectious diseases is more common. The incidence following measles is about 1 in 1000 (Miller, 1964). It occurs two to four days after the rash, and its course and prognosis are variable. Encephalitis is slightly less frequent after varicella and follows a relatively benign course, often with cerebellar ataxia.

Immunization

Since the publication of a report suggesting an association between pertussis vaccination and brain damage (Kulenkampff, 1974) there has been widespread publicity about the possible dangers of pertussis vaccine. The National Childhood Encephalopathy Study was established to assess the risks of serious neurological disorders associated with immunization. It concluded that the vast majority of cases of serious neurological illness in early childhood are attributable to causes other than immunization. However such illnesses were observed to occur more frequently than would be expected by chance within seven days, and in particular within 72 hours, of triple vaccine and within 7 to 14 days after measles vaccine (Miller *et al.*, 1981). Most affected children made a complete recovery. Their numbers, however, were small: of 1000 young children with serious neurological disease, only 32 previously normal children had received triple vaccine within seven days. Comparison of these cases with controls led to a calculated attributable risk of a serious neurological reaction to triple vaccine of 1 in 110 000, with a risk of persisting neurological damage one year later of 1 in 310 000 immunizations.

Convulsions and postictal states

Following a prolonged convulsion, consciousness may not be regained as a result of severe anoxic or ischaemic brain damage, which may be accompanied by cerebral oedema. Young children are particularly prone to convulse with a fever, and these convulsions may be prolonged.

Reye's syndrome

This rare condition is characterized by an acute and severe encephalopathy with diffuse fatty infiltration of the viscera, notably the liver. It was first described in Australia in 1963, but has been increasingly recognized ever since. It affects mainly children and adolescents,

Table 3   Clinical stages and liver function tests in Reye's syndrome (Lovejoy et al., 1974)

Stage	Clinical features	Blood ammonia	Serum transaminases
1	Vomiting, lethargy, drowsiness	↑	↑
2	Disorientation, aggression Hyper-reflexic, plantars upgoing Hyperventilation	↑↑	↑↑
3	Coma Upper midbrain dysfunction with decorticate posturing Fits Hyperventilation	↑↑	↑↑
4	Deepening coma Lower midbrain dysfunction with decerebrate posturing and loss of doll's eye response	↑	↑
5	Coma Medullary involvement with respiratory arrest, flaccidity and loss of reflexes	Normal	Normal

with an onset during the recovery phase from a mild upper respiratory infection, varicella or during influenza B epidemics. It remains uncertain whether aspirin ingestion is implicated in the pathogenesis of Reye's syndrome. The illness starts with vomiting, and is often accompanied by lethargy and drowsiness. These merge into signs of encephalopathy, with bizarre behaviour, often including agitation, aggression and hallucinations, progressing to coma. Fits are frequent, and hyperventilation a marked feature. It has proved useful to grade the severity of the disease and follow its progress using the criteria listed in Table 3.

Hepatic dysfunction can be demonstrated by the raised blood ammonia level which occurs early in the course of the illness, but returns to normal within 48-72 hours. Serum transaminases are raised but do not correlate with the severity of the illness. The prothrombin time is prolonged, but clinical jaundice is absent. Hypoglycaemia may be seen in young children. Blood gases show a respiratory alkalosis with a super-imposed metabolic acidosis. Reye's syndrome must be distinguished from more common conditions, particularly salicylate overdose, intracranial infection and post-anoxic encephalopathy. If the diagnosis is in doubt, a definitive diagnosis can be made on liver biopsy, when fatty infiltration can be demonstrated (Figures 2 and 3). A lumbar puncture may be required

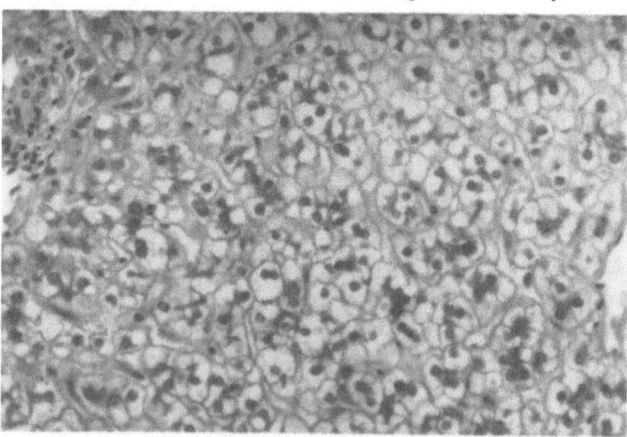

Figure 2 *Histology of the liver in Reye's syndrome. There are areas of vacuolation representing fat deposition and there is little inflammatory change (H and E stain)*

176

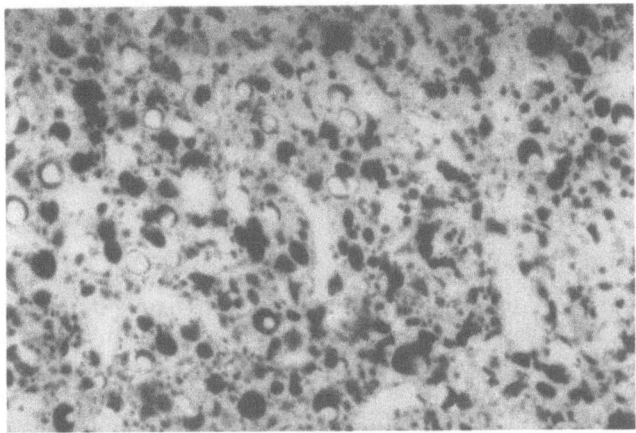

Figure 3 Histology of the liver in Reye's syndrome, showing microvesicular fatty infiltration. The globules representing fat can be identified with special stains (Oil red O stain)

in the early stages to rule out an intracranial infection, but it is best avoided as intracranial pressure is likely to be raised from cerebral oedema. The EEG is abnormal at all stages and mirrors the clinical severity.

Initial reports were of an 80 to 100% mortality and autopsy findings showed changes of gross cerebral oedema. Vigorous therapy to reduce cerebral oedema, introduced as early as possible, as well as intensive supportive care has resulted in a marked reduction in mortality. Other forms of treatment, in particular exchange transfusions and peritoneal dialysis, have been discontinued as they have been found to be ineffective.

Drugs

Drugs, in particular the tricyclic antidepressants and diphenoxylate (Lomotil) may cause fits and coma when taken in overdosage. Severe drug overdosage is seen less frequently in children than adults as most are the result of accidental rather than deliberate ingestion and it is uncommon for large quantities of drugs to be taken. Alcohol may precipitate an acute encephalopathy in children, together with profound hypoglycaemia. Lead encephalopathy is very rarely seen in England. (See Chapter 14 on Accidents and Poisoning.)

Head trauma

Head trauma is an important cause of coma. It is described on page 224.

Subdural haematoma

Subdural haematomas and effusions are seen mainly in the first two years of life. They are usually caused by trauma, but may follow meningitis or hypernatraemic dehydration. Nonaccidental injury either from direct trauma or vigorous shaking is an important cause to consider, and evidence of injury at other sites should be sought.

The clinical features of subdural haematomas and effusions in the infant are distinct from those seen in older children following trauma, when there is acute deterioration, progressive neurological dysfunction and focal signs. In infants, the signs tend to progress much more slowly, with nonspecific features of irritability, vomiting and lethargy, and it is only much later that convulsions and coma develop. The head may enlarge, the sutures become separated (Figure 4), the

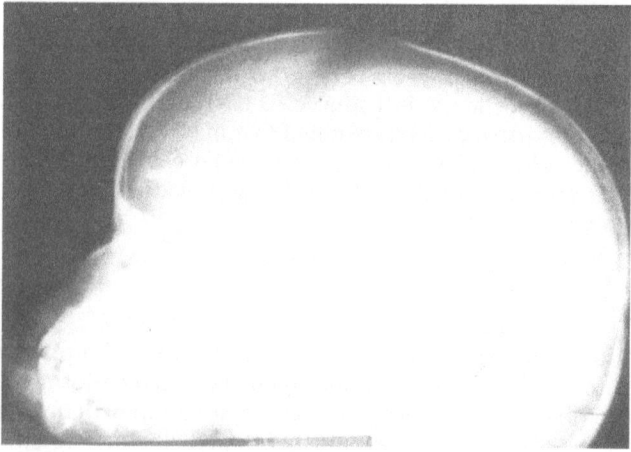

Figure 4   *An infant's skull radiograph showing separation of the sutures from raised intracranial pressure*

anterior fontanelle bulge and there may be retinal haemorrhages or abnormal neurological signs. Subdural haematomas may be detectable in infants by transillumination, ultrasound or CT scan. A neurosurgeon should be consulted about the subsequent management.

Hypertensive encephalopathy

Hypertensive encephalopathy (Figure 5) is much less common in children than adults. It is seen predominantly in children with acute glomerulonephritis and other renal disorders. In treating the hypertension a steady and gradual reduction in the blood pressure is the

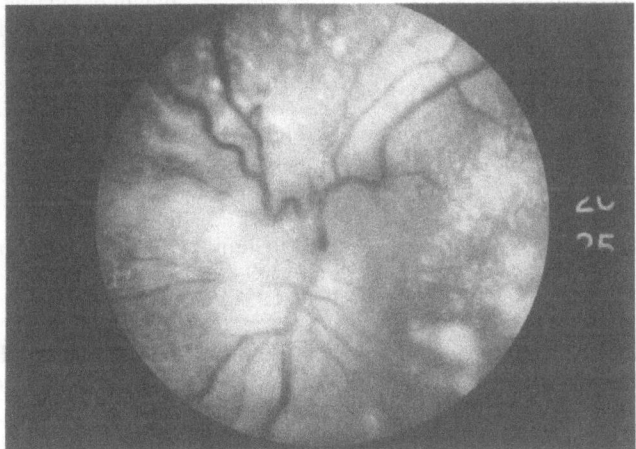

Figure 5   *Hypertensive retinopathy in a seven-year-old boy with renal disease*

aim. Precipitous falls may further compromise the blood flow through vessels which have been damaged by vasculitis secondary to the hypertension. The vessels of the retina, spinal cord and kidney are particularly at risk. There are several drugs available to use in severe hypertension (Table 4) but all have some disadvantages.

Post-anoxic encephalopathy

Children may suffer from an encephalopathy following prolonged anoxia. This may follow a cardiorespiratory arrest of any cause, but

179

Table 4   Drugs for the treatment of severe hypertension

Drug	Dose	Use	Comments
Diazoxide	3–5 mg/kg i.v.	Very severe hypertension requiring immediate treatment	Fall in blood pressure may be very rapid. (Can cause occipital blindness)
			Becomes protein bound and must be injected rapidly. Causes hyperglycaemia.
Hydralazine	0.2–1 mg/kg i.v.	Useful in moderate to severe hypertension	Fall in blood pressure may be very rapid. May be useful intramuscularly as adjunct to oral drugs.
Sodium nitroprusside	$0.5\,\mu g/kg^{-1}\,min^{-1}$ starting dose, to $5\,\mu g\,kg^{-1}\,min^{-1}$ i.v.	Severe hypertensive crisis	Brief action Potent vasodilator, monitor BP continuously
Minoxidil	2.5 mg/12 h starting dose, to 40 mg/24 h p.o.	Oral therapy of severe hypertension	Hirsutism with long-term therapy

especially respiratory obstruction from epiglottitis, laryngotracheo-bronchitis or foreign bodies, suffocation or drowning. It may also be seen in infants with 'near-miss' sudden infant death, who are noted to be pale or blue and to have stopped breathing and are then resuscitated.

Assessment

A physical examination and neurological assessment should be performed as soon as the child's respiratory and cardiovascular status are stable. Dehydration would suggest diabetes mellitus, severe gastroenteritis, peritonitis, intestinal obstruction or a salt-losing crisis. Hyperventilation is seen in diabetes mellitus, salicylate overdosage, hypernatraemic dehydration, Reye's syndrome, renal failure and in some of the inherited metabolic disorders. The level of consciousness must be determined and can be documented using a coma scale (Table 5) which should be modified according to the child's age.

Table 5   Coma scale (Teasdale and Jennett, 1974)

Eyes open	Best verbal response	Best motor response
Spontaneously	Oriented	Obeys commands
To speech	Confused	Localizes pain
To pain	Inappropriate words	Flexion to pain
None	Incomprehensible sounds	Extension to pain
	None	None

The neurological assessment should be directed towards evidence of an expanding cerebral hemisphere lesion and brainstem damage as these require urgent medical or neurosurgical treatment. Evidence needs to be sought of raised intracranial pressure, which may represent an expanding mass or obstruction of the CSF pathways. In an infant, the fontanelle may be tense, the sutures separated, and the scalp veins prominent. The head circumference may have increased rapidly and papilloedema is occasionally present. In an older child papilloedema suggests raised intracranial pressure and this may be accompanied by a slow pulse and raised blood pressure. However, papilloedema is frequently absent in spite of there being raised intracranial pressure. The pupil size and responsiveness to light needs to be checked. The presence of a unilateral dilated pupil with an impaired response to light indicates a third nerve palsy and implies temporal lobe herniation. Abnormalities of eye movements can be tested by rolling the head from side to side. (This should not be performed after trauma in case there is damage to the cervical spine.) Normally when the head of an unconscious person is moved to one side there is counterrolling of the eyes to the other side (doll's eye movements) but these movements may be dysconjugate, lost unilaterally or absent with brainstem lesions. A persistent hemiparesis, which may be detected by asymmetry of tone and reflexes, or an asymmetric response to a painful stimulus suggests that there may be a cerebral hemisphere lesion causing coma by brainstem compression.

Investigations

When a child in coma is first seen the cause may be suggested by the history and examination and the investigations selected accordingly (Table 6). Hypoglycaemia is the most treatable cause of coma; a

Table 6   **Investigations which may be required in a patient in coma**

Blood	Lumbar puncture
Full blood count	If indicated
Urea and electrolytes, osmolality	Blood
Blood glucose, calcium	Liver function tests
Blood gases	Ammonia
Blood culture	Viral titres
Clotting screen	Toxic screen of blood, urine and
Urine	gastric aspirate
MSU	Skull, spine and chest radiographs
Electrolytes and osmolality	CT scan
Test with Phenistix for salicylates	EEG

Dextrostix should be done immediately and the child treated if blood glucose is low. A confirmatory blood glucose is a useful check. Hypoglycaemia will not only be seen in children with diabetes mellitus, but also following alcohol ingestion, salicylate overdosage, in Reye's syndrome and some inherited metabolic diseases such as galactosaemia. In any child with fever and neck stiffness a lumbar puncture must be performed immediately. If there is papilloedema only a few drops of CSF should be taken. If any signs of coning develop during the procedure it has been suggested that 0.9% saline should be injected intrathecally to replace the fluid removed and intravenous mannitol given to reduce the cerebral oedema. Evidence of brain herniation at presentation is a contraindication to lumbar puncture but parenteral antibiotics as for bacterial meningitis should be started immediately if the child is febrile and has neck stiffness even if this reduces the chance of culturing an organism from the CSF later. A lumbar puncture is best avoided after a head injury or in Reye's syndrome. If there is raised intracranial pressure or focal neurological signs in the absence of a fever and neck stiffness an urgent CT scan will be needed. The CT scan is useful to demonstrate haemorrhage, an abscess, cerebral oedema, a tumour or focal necrosis of the temporal lobes in herpes simplex encephalitis.

Management

Respiratory support will be required if there is evidence of respiratory failure, irregular breathing or apnoeic attacks. Hypoventilation with retention of carbon dioxide must be avoided as it will increase cerebral congestion.

Cerebral oedema should be anticipated after a prolonged convulsion, following a respiratory arrest, any prolonged period of anoxia and in Reye's syndrome. It is also seen to a variable degree in meningitis and encephalitis. There are many measures available to reduce cerebral oedema, but it is impossible to make a rational selection of them and they are usually used empirically (Table 7). The

Table 7 Measures available to reduce cerebral oedema

Fluid restriction
One-third to two-thirds of maintenance fluids

Steroids
Dexamethasone 0.2 mg/kg i.v., then 0.25 to 0.5 mg kg^{-1} (24 h)$^{-1}$

Osmotic diuresis
Mannitol 0.5 to 1 g/kg given intravenously over 20 minutes

Hyperventilation
Reduce $Paco_2$ to 3.5 to 4 kPa (25-30 mmHg)

Barbiturates
Sodium thiopentone 30mg/kg as loading dose followed by
3 to 10 mg kg^{-1} h^{-1}

Hypothermia
Core temperature lowered to 32 °C

easiest is to restrict fluid intake to one-third to two-thirds maintenance and this will also counteract inappropriate secretion of ADH. If the patient is put on a ventilator hyperventilation can be employed, maintaining the $Paco_2$ at 3.5 to 4 kPa (25 to 30 mmHg) and ensuring adequate oxygenation. Any further reduction in the $Paco_2$ may reduce the pH of the CSF excessively and may itself cause an encephalopathy. Dexamethasone (Decadron) is known to disperse oedema around a tumour or abscess but there is doubt about its efficacy in oedema of other causes. Osmotic agents, particularly mannitol, act more quickly but can be dangerous if the child's serum osmolality is already very high, can result in severe overload if the child is in renal failure and there may be marked rebound after the infusion. Other methods of treatment include hypothermia and barbiturate therapy, which may reduce cerebral oxygen consumption and cerebral blood flow. The effect of these modes of therapy is unpredictable and means that the patient's clinical condition becomes very difficult to evaluate and he is totally dependent on artificial support. Various intracranial pressure monitors are available, but they are all invasive and have their own complications. They are available only in a few specialized centres and should be used on carefully selected patients.

Very severe cerebral oedema is usually encountered in Reye's syndrome, and the current trend in many units (Boutros *et al.*, 1980) is for endotracheal intubation at an early stage with hyperventilation, muscle relaxants and sedation. Fluids are severely restricted, and dexamethasone often given. Intracranial pressure monitoring may be employed and if the pressure remains high hypothermia and if necessary barbiturate therapy instituted. Mannitol is used for any sudden increases in pressure. A marked reduction in mortality and morbidity is reported.

All patients in coma require obsessional supportive care in an intensive care unit. The pulse, respiratory rate, temperature and blood pressure should be monitored continuously, and the level of consciousness, pupil size and responsiveness to light repeatedly assessed. The fluid balance, serum and urine electrolytes and osmolality, blood gases, haemoglobin, blood glucose and calcium levels will need to be measured regularly. This will often require an arterial line for repeated blood gases and continuous recording of the arterial blood pressure and a CVP line. In addition, attention needs to be paid to the prevention of gastric erosions, positional deformities and nutritional support. Amidst all the technology that is required, explanation and support for the child's parents and family must not be forgotten.

References

Boutros, A. R., Esfandiari, S., Orlowski, J. P. and Smith, O. S. (1980), *Pediatr. Clin. N. Am.*, **27**, 3, 539.

Kulenkampff, M., Schwartzmann, J.S. and Wilson, J. (1974), *Arch. Dis. Child.*, **49**, 46.

Lovejoy, F.H., Bresnan, J.J., Lombroso, C.T. and Smith, A.L. (1974), *Am. J. Dis. Child.*, **128**, 36.

Miller, D.L. (1964), *Br. Med. J.*, **2**, 75.

Miller, D.L., Ross, E.M., Alderslade, R., Bellman, M.H. and Rawson, N.S.B. (1981), *Br. Med. J.*, **282**, 1595.

Teasdale, G. and Jennett, B. (1974), *Lancet*, **2**, 81.

Whitley, R.J., Soong, S.J., Dolin, R., Galasso, G. J., Chlien, L. T. and Alford, C.A. (1977), *N. Engl. J. Med.*, **297**, 289.

Further reading

Weiner, H.L., Bresnan, M.J. and Levitt, L.P. (1977). *Paediatric Neurology for the House Officer*, Williams and Wilkins Co., Baltimore.

CHAPTER 11

Shock

When the blood flow is unable to meet the metabolic demands of the body's tissues a patient becomes shocked. The clinical features arise from the body's efforts to compensate for this circulatory failure. In children this compensation may be very effective and in the early stages it may be difficult to appreciate that the child is in shock until his condition suddenly and dramatically deteriorates. It is important to diagnose shock in its early stages when it is still reversible and amenable to treatment. The early signs are an anxious, irritable child with tachycardia and pale, cool, clammy extremities. The child may not yet be hypotensive, but the true severity of the illness may be gauged from a history of marked fluid loss or if the child is clinically severely dehydrated. The measurement of the difference between the central and peripheral temperature using a rectal probe and a probe attached to the big toe is helpful in assessing tissue perfusion, provided the child is in a warm environment (Aynsley-Green and Pickering, 1974). The temperature gap should not be more than 2 °C, and the renal output often falls when the temperature gap is 6 °C or more which is frequently before a detectable fall in the blood pressure. If the condition progresses, the child becomes lethargic, tachypnoeic, hypotensive with weak peripheral pulses, oliguric and develops a metabolic acidosis. The temperature may be elevated, depressed or unstable. Finally there may be coma, irregular respirations or cardiorespiratory arrest.

Aetiology

Shock is conventionally sub-divided according to its aetiology. It may be hypovolaemic, cardiogenic or from sepsis or anaphylaxis (Figure 1).

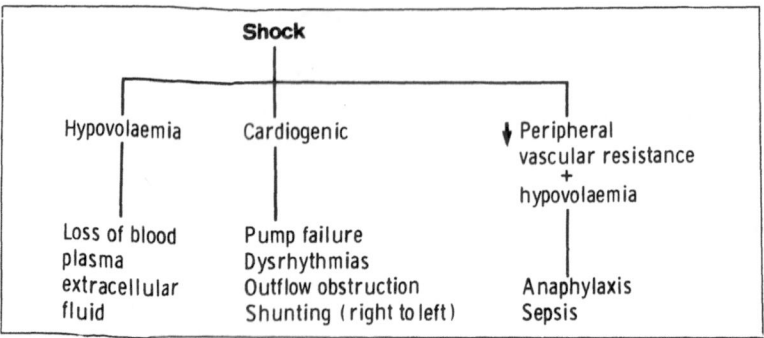

Figure 1   *The aetiology of shock*

Hypovolaemia is by far the commonest cause, where there is a loss of circulating blood volume from the loss of extracellular fluid, blood or plasma. Important causes are fluid and electrolyte loss from diarrhoea or diabetic ketoacidosis, blood loss from trauma or gastrointestinal bleeding and plasma loss from burns and peritonitis (Table 1).

Cardiogenic shock is unusual in paediatrics. Primary pump failure is rare but may occur with myocarditis, sepsis, in renal failure or

Table 1   Causes of hypovolaemia

Fluid and electrolyte loss
Diarrhoea and vomiting
Diabetic ketoacidosis

Blood loss
Trauma
Gastrointestinal bleeding

Plasma loss
Burns
Peritonitis and intestinal obstruction
Capillary leak from acidosis and sepsis
Hypoproteinaemia

following cardiac surgery. Outflow obstruction may be seen in congenital heart disease, with a tension pneumothorax or a pericardial effusion.

Marked reduction in peripheral vascular resistance with an increase in the venous capacitance is seen in septic shock and anaphylaxis. In septic shock there is also volume depletion and there may be cardiogenic shock.

Management

In all cases the priority is to ensure an adequate airway and give oxygen and artificial ventilation if required. A suitable line for intravenous infusion must be rapidly established, either by percutaneous puncture, or occasionally via a cut down (see page 288) and infusion 288) provided one is skilled in this technique. A low CVP suggests fluid for infusion continues to be controversial. Of the colloids, pooled plasma has a small but definite risk of transfusion hepatitis and has largely been replaced by purified protein fraction (PPF). The main alternatives to plasma preparations for volume expansion are Haemaccel, the dextrans and hydroethyl starches (Hetaplas). Haemaccel, a degraded gelatin solution, has the advantage over the dextrans that it does not interfere with the cross-matching of blood or impair blood coagulation. Plasma protein fraction is always immediately available and is widely used in severe cases of shock for initial vascular expansion. Thereafter, the choice of infusion will depend on the fluid lost.

Blood must be given to replace blood loss, and plasma protein fraction continued for plasma loss as in burns or from capillary leakage from severe metabolic acidosis or sepsis.

Hypovolaemic shock

An outline of the initial management of shock is shown in Figure 2. Initially 10 ml/kg of a plasma expander is given rapidly. A repeat infusion of fluid is given if necessary as judged by the clinical response and the calculated fluid deficit. If the child is clearly still volume depleted, a further bolus may be required, otherwise the infusion rate can be changed to $10 \, \text{ml} \, \text{kg}^{-1} \, \text{h}^{-1}$.

Improvement may be judged by increase in tissue perfusion, pulse

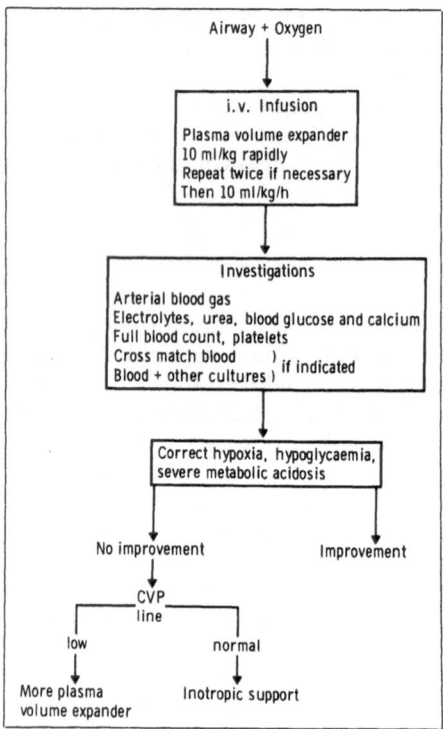

Figure 2   *An outline of the management of shock*

rate, blood pressure and in the central-peripheral temperature difference. An adequate urine output ($0.5\,\text{ml kg}^{-1}\,\text{h}^{-1}$ or $> 10\,\text{ml m}^{-2}\,\text{h}^{-1}$) suggests both an adequate renal blood flow and cardiac output. Continued oliguria may result from renal hypoperfusion from inadequately corrected hypovolaemia or may be a sign of acute renal failure. The investigations listed in Figure 2 will need to be performed urgently, and an estimate of the blood glucose performed at the bedside with a Dextrostix or a BM-Test-Glycemie '20-800' strip. Arterial blood gases will reflect the adequacy of ventilation and degree of metabolic acidosis. Blood and other cultures will need to be taken and broad spectrum antibiotics started if sepsis is suspected. The child should be transferred to the intensive care unit.

Most children will improve with expansion of their plasma volume, but if this has not been the case a CVP line is extremely helpful to monitor subsequent fluid therapy. One or more central lines can usually be rapidly inserted via the right internal jugular vein (see p. 288) provided one is skilled in this technique. A low CVP suggests that the hypovolaemia has not been corrected and more plasma volume expansion is indicated. Although the normal range for the CVP (5-10 cm of water) is a useful guide, the optimal pressure for an individual patient has to be assessed from the response to further infusions. Attention also needs to be paid to the correction of hypoxia, abnormalities of acid-base balance, electrolytes, hypoglycaemia and hypocalcaemia. The metabolic acidosis will resolve with improvement in tissue perfusion, but if very severe may be partially and slowly corrected with sodium bicarbonate watching that the child does not become sodium overloaded or hypokalaemic. Potassium should never be added to the intravenous infusion until an adequate urine flow has been established and the plasma potassium estimated.

Rarely, in spite of the correction of hypovolaemia, the patient will remain hypotensive with poor skin perfusion and oliguria suggesting a falling cardiac output from myocardial dysfunction. Further circulatory support to increase the cardiac output will need to be considered (Figure 3). In infants the cardiac output is highly dependent on the heart rate and only a small reduction is needed to produce a large reduction in cardiac output. Initial cardiovascular support should be with an agent with a significant chronotropic effect. Of the sympathomimetic agents isoprenaline (isoproterenol) is the most

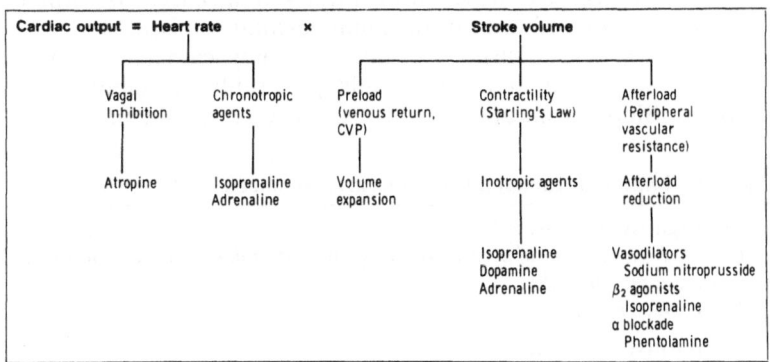

Figure 3   *Agents to increase cardiac output*

191

widely used. Dopamine in low dosage may be given in addition to isoprenaline or sometimes on its own, to provide additional inotropic support and for its specific action in increasing renal blood flow. Dobutamine is an almost pure inotropic agent with little effect on the blood vessels. The dosages of these agents are adjusted according to the clinical response. Sometimes after-load reduction, for example with sodium nitroprusside or α-blockers like chlorpromazine or phenoxybenzamine is used when there is pump failure with elevated peripheral vascular resistance. Peripheral vasodilatation can be useful to relieve the continuing metabolic acidosis and other metabolic consequences of severe peripheral vasoconstriction which may continue even though the cardiac output has increased. However the effects of these agents cannot be predicted with any accuracy. If these or any of the sympathomimetic agents are given, the CVP, blood pressure and heart rate must be closely monitored as they may profoundly alter the peripheral vascular resistance.

Septic shock

Bacterial pathogens, especially the Gram-negative organisms, are the most frequent cause of septic shock (Table 2). In contrast to hypovolaemic shock, these patients may initially have warm peripheries. Purpura are often seen with meningococcal septicaemia. Rarely the characteristic green skin lesions of pseudomonas septicaemia are seen. There may be disseminated intravascular coagulation (DIC) with petechiae and bleeding, especially from puncture sites. Patients at particular risk are those with central venous catheters, urinary tract obstruction or burns, or the immune-compromised.

If septic shock is suspected, any indwelling catheters or other potential sources of infection should preferably be removed and cultured. Blood, urine and, if indicated, the CSF should be cultured,

Table 2   Important bacterial pathogens in septic shock

Gram-negative organisms
  E. coli, *Klebsiella aerobacter*, *Proteus* group, *Pseudomonas aeruginosa*
  Neiserria meningitidis
  Bacteroides species

Gram-positive organisms
  Clostridia, staphylococci, streptococci and pneumococci

and antibiotics given. For meningococcal septicaemia, high dose intravenous penicillin is the drug of choice, otherwise broad spectrum antibiotics must be given until the organism has been identified. Suitable combinations depend on the clinical situation but include gentamicin together with azlocillin, cloxacillin or cefuroxime. If it is thought that anaerobic organisms are a likely pathogen, metronidazole is added.

Infusion of plasma volume expander and the many supportive measures described in hypovolaemic shock will be required. In addition steroids in pharmacological doses are often advocated. Fresh frozen plasma is usually given to provide clotting factors. If DIC is present, treatment is primarily of the underlying infection. Heparin would appear to be rarely indicated but may be used when there is serious bleeding or overt thrombotic complications. It is best given as a continuous infusion ($25\,U\,kg^{-1}\,h^{-1}$).

Anaphylaxis

Mild allergic reactions presenting with urticaria are common. The allergens most frequently identified are listed in Table 3, but often none is identified. Symptomatic treatment for the itching with an antihistamine such as diphenhydramine (Benedryl) or chlorpheniramine (Piriton) may be given.

Severe systemic anaphylaxis is rare but needs urgent treatment as it is life-threatening from laryngeal oedema, bronchospasm, shock and cardiorespiratory arrest. These serious attacks mostly occur

Table 3   Some important allergens causing anaphylaxis

Drugs
   Penicillin
   Asparaginase
   Local anaesthetics
   Contrast media for radiological investigations
Desensitization injections, e.g. for hay fever
Immune sera, e.g. diphtheria, tetanus, antilymptocyte serum, gamma
   globulin
Blood transfusion
Food allergies
   milk, egg, shellfish, nuts
Insect stings
   bees, wasps

193

minutes after a drug has been administered or following an insect bite. Immediate therapy has been summarized in Table 4. An adequate airway must be ensured, oxygen given together with artificial ventilation if necessary. Adrenaline must be injected immediately, and as absorption from a subcutaneous injection may be unreliable and delayed, it is probably better to give it by slow intravenous injection with ECG monitoring. In the less severe attack, the adrenaline can be given subcutaneously. A tourniquet should be placed proximal to the site of an injection or insect bite. In anaphylactic shock there is extreme peripheral vasodilatation with moderate myocardial depression. Adrenaline is the drug of choice as it will arrest the allergic process, and is a peripheral vasoconstrictor as well as having inotropic properties. Aminophylline is given if there is bronchospasm. Antihistamines are given intravenously together with steroids to ameliorate symptoms over the next 24 hours.

Table 4 Treatment of life-threatening anaphylaxis

Immediate
  Adequate airway, oxygen, IPPV if necessary
  Adrenaline
    intravenously 1:10000 (0.1 mg/ml)
                0.1 ml/kg slowly, repeat in 5 min if necessary
    subcutaneous 1:1000 (1 mg/ml)
                0.01 ml/kg, repeat in 5 min if necessary, to max. total
                dose of 0.5 ml

Subsequent
  Plasma volume expander ± sympathomimetic agents
  Aminophylline
    Loading dose 5-6 mg/kg, then $1\,mg\,kg^{-1}\,h^{-1}$ by continuous infusion
  Antihistamine
    Chlorpheniramine (Piriton) i.v. 0.25 mg/kg to maximum dose of 10 mg
  Steroids
    Hydrocortisone 100-200 mg i.v.

References and further reading

Aynsley-Green, A. and Pickering, D. (1974). Use of central and peripheral temperature measurements in care of the critically ill child. *Arch. Dis. Child.*, **49**, 477.
Crane, R.K. (1980). Acute circulatory failure in children. *Pediatr. Clin. N. Am.*, **27**, 3, 525.

CHAPTER 12

Disorders of the kidney and urinary tract

In this chapter the complications of the nephrotic syndrome will be described and an outline given of the management of acute renal failure, the haemolytic–uraemic syndrome and urinary tract infection.

Nephrotic syndrome

In the nephrotic syndrome, there is gross proteinuria ($>0.05\,\mathrm{g\,kg^{-1}}$ $(24\,\mathrm{h})^{-1}$ or $>40\,\mathrm{mg\,m^{-2}\,h^{-1}}$), hypoalbuminaemia (plasma albumin $<25\,\mathrm{g/l}$, $2.5\,\mathrm{g}/100\,\mathrm{ml}$) and oedema. The initial presentation is usually with oedema. Most of these children have periorbital oedema (Figure 1) and many have oedema of the legs, the scrotum and there may be ascites. Children with nephrotic syndrome are at particular risk from hypovolaemia, thromboses and infection and these complications are described. An account of the overall management of the nephrotic syndrome will not be given.

Hypovolaemia

In the nephrotic syndrome fluid shifts from the intravascular to the extravascular compartment. This is because of the low plasma oncotic pressure resulting from the hypoproteinaemia. Symptomatic hypovolaemia occurs if the fluid shift is large and is usually seen at initial presentation or early in relapse. It will be exacerbated by any

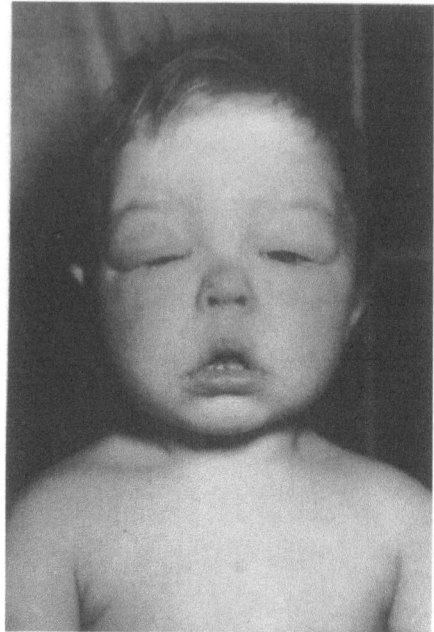

Figure 1   *Gross periorbital oedema in a boy with nephrotic syndrome*

additional losses of fluid from the intravascular compartment from diarrhoea, vomiting or after giving diuretics. These children often complain of abdominal pain and any child with nephrotic syndrome who develops this symptom needs to be carefully assessed. Those with hypovolaemia may also feel faint or generally unwell.

Hypovolaemia can be detected by measuring the haematocrit or Hb. It is suggested if the haematocrit is greater than 48% or by a rapid rise in haematocrit (Table 1). Another helpful indicator is a urine sodium concentration of less than 5 mmol/l. There may be evidence of peripheral circulatory failure but the pulse rate and blood

Table 1   Indications for treatment of hypovolaemia

Haematocrit > 48% or Hb > 16 g/100 ml
Rapid rise in haematocrit > 6% or more than 2 g/100 ml in the Hb
Peripheral circulatory failure

pressure are often maintained within the normal range by peripheral vasoconstriction. The blood pressure may even be raised due to increased renin production. Hyponatraemia may be present from drinking water in excess of salt or may be an artefact from the hyperlipidaemia. Rarely, there may be acute tubular necrosis from severe hypovolaemia, but this can be identified by examining the quality of the urine passed (Table 3). The treatment of hypovolaemia is to re-expand the plasma volume with salt-poor albumin (1 g/kg) and monitor the response by measuring the pulse, respiratory rate and blood pressure, the rate of urine production and the central-peripheral temperature gap. A CVP line is useful in the presence of renal failure. If the child is hyponatraemic plasma may be preferred to salt-poor albumin, to avoid exacerbating hyponatraemia, but care needs to be taken not to overload the circulation as there will also be fluid returning from the extracellular compartment. Diuretics should preferably be avoided in the early stages of relapse unless a plasma volume expander is given first.

Thromboses

Thromboses, usually venous but occasionally arterial, can have a high morbidity or be fatal. They arise from a combination of hyperviscosity, from hypovolaemia, and abnormal clotting factors. Avoiding hypovolaemia and discouraging bed rest will help prevent thromboses.

Infection

Children with the nephrotic syndrome are particularly susceptible to infection. This susceptibility is enhanced if they are being treated with steroids or other immunosuppressive agents. The organism classically involved is the pneumococcus causing especially primary pneumococcal peritonitis and cellulitis, but the Gram-negative organisms are equally important. It has already been stressed that abdominal pain is an important symptom in children with nephrotic syndrome as it may signal hypovolaemia. Another important cause is primary peritonitis. If peritonitis is suspected it can be confirmed by aspirating, with a fine needle, a small volume of ascitic fluid and examining it by microscopy, culture and sensitivity or counter current immunoelectrophoresis. Because of the risk of cellulitis careful skin care is required of grossly oedematous parts, especially the scrotum, and of the sites of intravenous infusions. Penicillin is often given prophylactically whilst there is proteinuria.

Acute renal failure

Acute renal failure in children is uncommon. There is usually oliguria, with less than $0.5 \, ml \, kg^{-1} \, h^{-1} \, (300 \, ml \, m^{-2} \, (24 \, h)^{-1})$ of urine. In acute renal failure the kidney is suddenly unable to maintain normal renal function. This failure of renal function may be due to inadequate renal blood flow (pre-renal), damage to the kidneys themselves (renal), or from obstruction to the excretion of urine (post-renal) (Table 2).

Table 2   Classification of acute renal failure

Pre-renal	Renal	Post-renal
Hypovolaemia diarrhoea and vomiting burns acute haemorrhage nephrotic syndrome	Acute tubular nephropathy ischaemia, nephrotoxins	Obstructive lesions megacystis-mega-ureter posterior urethral valves stones
Circulatory failure septicaemia heart failure	Acute interstitial nephropathy drugs	
	Acute glomerulonephritis	
	Haemolytic-uraemic syndrome	
	Renal vein thrombosis	

Priorities in management are to distinguish pre-renal from renal failure, to exclude urinary obstruction and to rapidly treat pre-renal failure. The presence of any pre-existing renal disease will need to be established.

Pre-renal failure

Pre-renal failure is caused by renal hypoperfusion. It is by far the commonest cause of acute renal failure in children. It may follow

198

shock and is seen especially from hypovolaemia following profuse diarrhoea. Hypovolaemia must be urgently corrected by expansion of the vascular volume and this needs to be carefully monitored. Once oliguria has developed there is a risk that tubular damage has occurred, and this can be identified by examination of the blood and urine. In pre-renal failure the kidneys are still able to form urine with a high osmolality and a low concentration of sodium but if the tubules have been damaged this ability is lost (Table 3). If the child

Table 3   Investigations to distinguish pre-renal from renal failure

Measurement	Pre-renal	Renal
Urinary volume	$<0.5\,\mathrm{ml\,kg^{-1}\,h^{-1}}$	Variable
Urine osmolality (mosmol/kg)	>500	(use the urine to plasma osmolality ratio)
Urine : plasma osmolality ratio	>1.3	<1.1
Urinary Na (mmol/l)*	<10	>20
Urinary urea (mmol/l)	>250 ($>1500\,\mathrm{mg}/100\,\mathrm{ml}$)	<100 ($<600\,\mathrm{mg}/100\,\mathrm{ml}$)

* If loop diuretics have not been used.

remains oliguric in spite of adequate fluid replacement, it may be possible to increase urine output by giving large doses of frusemide intravenously (5–10 mg/kg). Mannitol is sometimes used but it has the disadvantage of causing circulatory overload if it is not excreted.

Renal failure

There are many different facets to the investigation and management of renal failure which will need to be done simultaneously. These children should be referred to a paediatric nephrology centre, especially if dialysis may be required. Some of the investigations which are likely to be needed are listed in Table 4, and the management of some of the specific problems listed in Table 5. Peritoneal rather than haemodialysis is usually the method of choice in the acute situation. It should be begun early rather than waiting for serious complications. It may be required for fluid overload manifest as pulmonary

Table 4 Some of the investigations and measurements in acute renal failure

Investigation	Comments
Blood: electrolytes, urea, osmolality, creatinine, acid–base balance, Ca, P, Mg, glucose alkaline phosphatase, protein	Required urgently, then serial measurements.
Urine: electrolytes, osmolality	Distinguish pre-renal from renal failure
protein	Heavy proteinuria, red blood cells,
microscopy	red cell or granular casts suggest renal disease
culture and sensitivity	Important to identify urinary tract infections
Full blood count, platelets	Identify anaemia and coagulation disorder,
Clotting studies, if indicated	especially in haemolytic uraemic syndrome
Blood cultures and other cultures	Septicaemia often present and must be identified
Radiographs: chest and abdomen wrist and hand	Identify renal osteodystrophy from pre-existing renal failure
Ultrasound Renal radio-isotope scans High dose IVU; MCU — as indicated	Identify cause of renal failure Must exclude obstructive causes
ECG	Monitor continuously Look for electrolyte abnormalities and conduction defects
Weight	Measure regularly as guide to fluid balance
Fluid balance	Meticulous record of input and output

Table 5 Outline of the management of acute renal failure

Pre-renal failure	Expansion of circulating volume with 20 ml/kg of blood, plasma or 0.9% saline.
Water overload	Frusemide 2–10 mg/kg i.v. Restrict fluid intake to fluid output + any extra losses (e.g. pyrexia) + minimum fluid requirement (basal insensible loss minus water of oxidation– 22 mg/kg from birth to 9 months falling to 18 ml/kg by 2 years and 9.5 ml/kg by 12 years). Dialysis
Pulmonary oedema	Frusemide i.v. and dialysis Intermittent positive pressure ventilation
Hypertension	Hydrallazine 0.5–1 mg/kg i.m. or i.v. Frusemide
Hyperkalaemia (plasma $K > 7$ mmol/l)	Sodium bicarbonate cautiously Calcium potassium exchange ⎫ temporary resin orally and rectally 1 g/kg ⎭ reduction 2 ml/kg of 2.5% calcium gluconate– temporarily opposes effect on heart Dialysis
Acidosis	Cautiously correct with sodium bicarbonate. Watch for Na overload or hypokalaemia
Convulsions	Diazepam 0.2 mg/kg i.v. Correct underlying cause
Infection	Important to identify. Ampicillin and cloxacillin if required in normal doses, gentamicin loading dose then increase time interval and monitor blood levels.
Prevent catabolism	Aim for energy intake to equal at least the basal requirements with first class protein intake of at least 1 g/kg.

oedema, or hypertension, hyperkalaemia or rapidly progressing azotaemia and acidosis. When to institute dialysis will also be influenced by the nature of the underlying disease. If expertly managed, the prognosis of acute renal failure in childhood is much better than in adults.

Haemolytic–uraemic syndrome

In the haemolytic–uraemic syndrome there is an acute onset of hae-molytic anaemia, thrombocytopenia and renal failure. It is rare and mainly affects pre-school children. The most common initial com-plaint is of vomiting and diarrhoea, which may contain blood. This is followed within the next two weeks by the child becoming pale, and developing haematuria and marked oliguria. Hypertension is common and the blood film shows microangiopathic haemolytic anaemia with many fragmented cells and thrombocytopenia. Other features at presentation may be irritability, convulsions and coma. Purpura may be present and the children are often oedematous. This syndrome seems to be the result of 'effective' prostacyclin deficiency. To try and replace this deficiency some centres have been giving daily infusions of fresh frozen plasma. Otherwise the management is of the renal failure and dialysis is often required. The anaemia may require blood transfusions. The mortality has been markedly reduced by improved management of the renal failure, but about 3-4% never recover renal function and about 15% later develop terminal renal insufficiency.

Urinary tract infection

Urinary tract infections are common in childhood. The risk of a newborn boy developing a urinary tract infection during childhood is about 1% and for a girl 3%. An accurate diagnosis of a urinary tract infection (UTI) must be made, not only to serve as a guide for appropriate antibiotic therapy, but to initiate investigations of the urinary tract and long-term follow-up which are important in iden-tifying underlying renal tract abnormalities and possibly prevent subsequent renal damage. Meticulous attention must be paid to the correct collection of urine specimens and to ensure that they are properly processed, otherwise incorrect diagnoses will be made and children subjected unnecessarily to further investigations. In babies, if organisms are cultured from a bag urine the diagnosis should be confirmed with a supra-pubic aspirate of urine (see page 292). A UTI is indicated by a pure growth of more than 10^9 organisms/l ($>100\,000$ organisms/ml) on a clean catch specimen, or any growth from a supra-pubic aspirate. In the sick child, microscopy of the urine for white cells and organisms is especially helpful, and may be the only guide if the child is already on antibiotics.

Clinical features

The older child may complain of dysuria or frequency. Other clinical features are abdominal pain, either acute or recurrent, loin pain or a fever. Dysuria is also seen in the acute urethral syndrome, from balanitis or acute vulvitis. Symptoms are much less specific in the young child. Acute symptoms are fever, febrile convulsions, vomiting or diarrhoea, or the presentation may be more chronic with poor feeding or failure to thrive. A sample of urine needs to be taken for microscopy and culture from every sick child. In the neonate about half are septicaemic. A fever may or may not be present, many have poor weight gain and some have prolonged jaundice.

Therapy

Drug sensitivities will serve as a guide in choosing an antibiotic. The commonest urinary pathogen is *E. coli* and then other normal bowel commensals. Antibiotics in full therapeutic dosage are usually given for ten days with a repeat MSU two to three days after therapy has begun and after a similar time interval following the completion of treatment. Co-trimoxazole is particularly useful, and other antibiotics often used are nitrofurantoin and nalidixic acid. Amoxycillin can be used but may induce resistant organisms. For the seriously ill child with septicaemia, intravenous gentamicin is the drug of choice, modifying the time interval between doses if renal function is compromised.

Investigations

Investigation of children who have had a single UTI shows that 10% have unsuspected and serious underlying urinary tract malformations and an additional 30-40% have vesicoureteric reflux (VUR) (Figure 2). It appears that renal scarring is especially likely in young children when there is a combination of infected urine and reflux, especially if there is intra-renal reflux. It may be possible to prevent renal scarring by ensuring that the urine remains free of infection and correcting any outflow obstruction.

There is no generally accepted plan of investigation. In the newborn good quality intravenous urograms (IVU) are difficult to obtain but ultrasound by experienced radiologists can be used to detect any

203

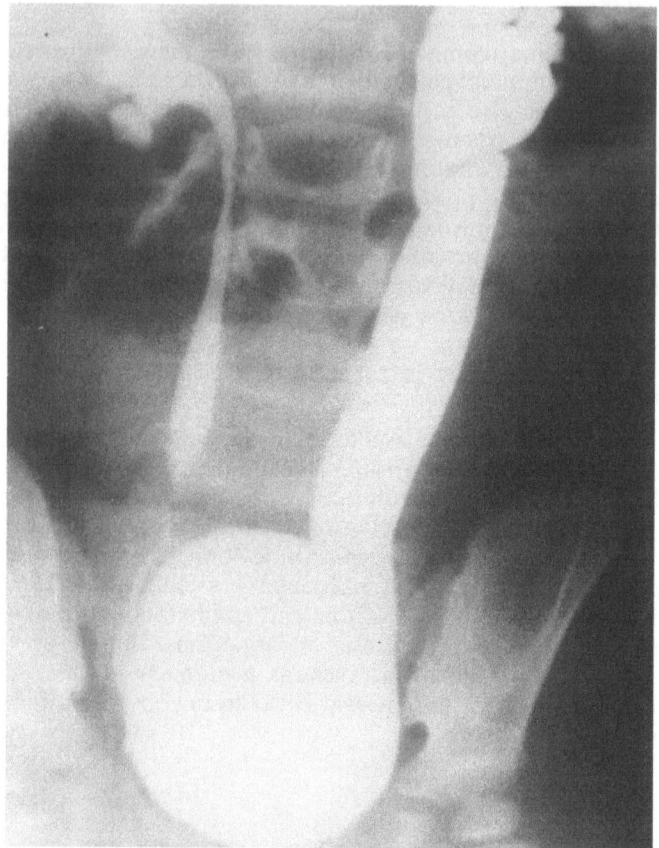

Figure 2 *A micturating cystourethrogram in a child who had a urinary tract infection. There is gross vesicoureteric reflex*

serious underlying structural abnormality. An IVU is indicated in every child with a UTI and in children with a clinical history suggestive of one. Serious renal scarring has usually occurred by the age of 5 years and a micturating cystourethrogram has been recommended to detect VUR in all children less than 5 years old, in those with any renal abnormalities or dilatation of the ureters on the IVU, or for recurrent urinary tract infections (Smellie, 1979). More recently, ultrasound and radio-isotope scanning have been introduced, but their place has yet to be clearly defined.

Follow-up

All children with a UTI should have regular MSUs and follow-up for a minimum of 2 years. Three-quarters of the girls will have a further UTI in that time, most in the first six months. Where there is VUR, many will resolve spontaneously but this depends partly on the severity of reflux. When it has been identified, depending on the age of the child and the degree of reflux, decisions will have to be made about starting long-term low dosage prophylactic antibiotics or surgical re-implantation of the ureters. The latter is usually reserved for gross reflux with widely dilated ureters in young children, fresh renal scarring, poor renal growth or recurrent infections in spite of antibiotics. Attention also needs to be paid to good personal hygiene and double micturition before going to bed to avoid leaving residual urine in the bladder.

References and Further Reading

Barratt, T.M. (1979), Nephrotic syndrome. In: *Paediatric Therapeutics*. Valman, H.B. (ed). Blackwell Scientific Publications, Oxford.

Chantler, C. (1979), Renal Failure in Childhood. In: *Renal Disease*. Black, D. and Jones, N.F. (eds). Blackwell Scientific Publications, Oxford.

Smellie, J.M. (1979). Management of urinary tract infection. In: *Paediatric Therapeutics*. Valman, H.B. (ed). Blackwell Scientific Publications, Oxford.

CHAPTER 13

Cardiovascular emergencies

The spectrum of cardiovascular disease in children is very different from that of adults. It comprises almost exclusively congenital disorders and their complications. Ischaemic heart disease is extremely rare in this age group, although myocardial ischaemic damage is occasionally seen in the newborn following severe hypoxia. As rheumatic fever is now uncommon in Britain acquired heart disease has become a relatively minor problem. The incidence of congenital heart disorders is high at 8-10 per 1000 births. They cover a wide range of severity. Some disorders present acutely in the neonatal period or infancy whilst others have a more chronic presentation and may be detected in asymtomatic children on hearing a heart murmur. Infants and babies with severe heart disease develop cyanosis, heart failure or a combination of these. The age of the child is helpful in assessing the most likely underlying cause (Figure 1). The commonest cardiac lesions presenting in the first week of life are listed in Table 1.

Cyanosis

The clinical identification of cyanosis is not reliable. Cyanosis can be detected clinically only when there is 5 g/dl of circulating reduced haemoglobin and is therefore dependent on the patient's haemoglobin concentration. In some forms of complex cyanotic heart disease where there is a right-to-left shunt but increased pulmonary

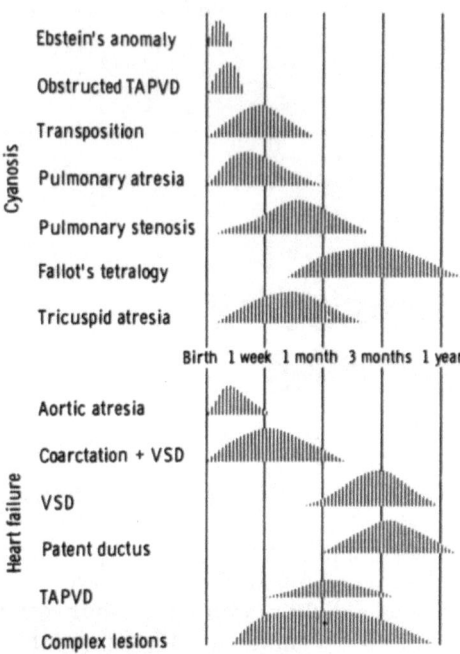

Figure 1 *The age of onset of symptoms from cardiac disease during the first year of life. Reproduced with permission from Jordan and Scott, 1981*

Table 1 Cardiac lesions which commonly present in the first week of life

Cyanosis	Heart failure	Cyanosis and heart failure
Transposition of the great arteries	Hypoplastic left heart syndrome	Transposition of the great arteries
Univentricular heart with absent atrio-ventricular connexion	Coarctation of the aorta or interrupted aortic arch	Total anomalous pulmonary venous drainage
(Tricuspid atresia)	Complex lesions	Complex lesions
Pulmonary atresia		
Total anomalous pulmonary venous drainage		

blood flow (as in some types of univentricular hearts), the oxygen saturation of the blood may be sufficient for cyanosis to be undetectable. Cyanosis is not always indicative of cyanotic heart disease as children with acyanotic heart disease may become cyanosed if they develop heart failure or a chest infection.

True central cyanosis must be differentiated from peripheral cyanosis, which is common in the newborn, from the plethoric appearance of the polycythaemic infant and rarely from methaemoglobinaemia.

Differentiating cardiac from non-cardiac causes of cyanosis (Table 2) can be difficult in the newborn. The main group of non-cardiac

Table 2   Causes of central cyanosis in the newborn

Cardiac
Respiratory
    Respiratory distress syndrome
    Pneumonia
    Aspiration
    Pneumothorax
    Diaphragmatic hernia
    Persistent fetal circulation
Choanal atresia
Central nervous system damage

disorders to consider is respiratory, especially the respiratory distress syndrome in the preterm infant, pneumonia and aspiration. Persistant fetal circulation, when the pulmonary vascular resistance remains high resulting in right-to-left shunting across the foramen ovale and ductus arteriosus, can be particularly difficult to differentiate. Respiratory distress from a pneumothorax or diaphragmatic hernia will be diagnosed from the chest radiograph. In choanal atresia there is difficulty breathing and cyanosis from birth, but it is relieved by breathing through the mouth with the help of an oral airway. Cyanosis may also be seen from central nervous system damage in association with apnoea or irregular respirations and abnormal neurological signs.

Cyanotic heart disease occurs with right-to-left shunting of blood and reduced pulmonary blood flow, in the presence of complete transposition of the great arteries or if there is common mixing of the pulmonary and systemic venous return.

Clinical examination

Clinical examination of the baby may reveal evidence of cardiac disease. Abnormal precordial motion may be either seen or felt. There may be abnormalities of the heart sounds, especially the second, and in the way in which its components split but this may be difficult to discern in the neonate as the heart rate is so rapid. A heart murmur may be heard. The peripheral arterial pulses or the blood pressure may be abnormal. However, there may not be any specific abnormalities of the cardiovascular system on physical examination alone, and in particular no heart murmurs.

Investigations

The investigations required are a chest radiograph, ECG, the blood pressure and the hyperoxia test (nitrogen washout test). In addition the blood glucose, calcium and electrolytes will need to be checked. The features which need to be considered on the chest radiograph are the position and size of the heart and the cardiac silhouette. Most important is the state of the pulmonary vasculature, and it has to be decided if the vascular markings in the peripheral lung fields are normal, increased (pulmonary plethora) or decreased (pulmonary oligaemia). Additional problems in the neonate are that it can be difficult to obtain optimally orientated radiographs, the thymus may be very large which may give a spurious appearance of cardiomegaly and it may not be easy to assess the pulmonary vasculature as the variation in the normal is so wide at this age. The ECG may show abnormalities of the axis, rate or rhythm and of atrial or ventricular hypertrophy or dominance. (Further details are given in the appendix.) On the basis of only the physical examination, chest radiograph and ECG it is often not possible to make a specific anatomical diagnosis with certainty, but rather to establish that the baby has congenital heart disease. The hyperoxia test (Jones, 1976) is helpful in distinguishing if the cyanosis is cardiac or non-cardiac in origin. The baby is placed in a head box in 100% oxygen for 10 minutes, and an arterial sample, preferably from the right radial artery, as it is preductal, is taken. Care must be taken to ensure that the baby remains in 100% oxygen whilst the sample is taken. Cyanotic heart disease is excluded if the arterial oxygen is above 33 kPa (250 mmHg) and is unlikely if it is above 21 kPa (160 mmHg). If the baby is breathing normally, a Pa_2 less than 13 kPa (100 mmHg) strongly suggests cyanotic heart disease but if the Pa_2 is less than 4 kPa (30 mmHg) complete transposition of the great arteries is the most likely diagnosis. If the baby is tachypnoeic, the low Pa_2 may also be from severe lung disease (in which case the $PaCO_2$ may be raised), or from persistent fetal circulation (when the second heart sound is single and loud).

Management

Neonates with cyanotic congenital heart disease need to be managed in a paediatric cardiology centre, where echocardiography and cardiac catheterization are available and surgery can be performed if necessary. The baby may need transferring and this should be arranged promptly. Prior to transfer the baby's breathing needs to be assessed and assisted ventilation instituted if necessary. Most of these babies can be nursed in 30-40% oxygen. A severe metabolic acidosis will need to be partially corrected. These babies are prone to hypothermia and this should be prevented. It is also important to consider whether to start a prostaglandin infusion.

Table 3   Prostaglandin infusion

(a) *Indications*
     Ductus dependent pulmonary blood flow
          Pulmonary atresia or critical pulmonary stenosis
          Severe tetralogy of Fallot
          Ebstein's anomaly
     Ductus dependent aortic blood flow
          Coarctation of the aorta or interrupted aortic arch

(b) *Dose*
     Prostaglandin E_1 or E_2 0.05-0.1 μg kg^{-1} min^{-1} by continuous i.v. infusion.

(c) *Side-effects*
          Apnoea
          Hypotension
          Pyrexia
          Muscle twitching
          Irritability
          Residual ductal patency (in 5%)

Prostaglandins will keep the ductus patent and are indicated if there is ductus dependent pulmonary or aortic blood flow. A prostaglandin infusion should be started in any baby where the lung fields are oligaemic on the chest radiograph or if there is severe hypoxia or acidosis associated with poor cardiac output. If in doubt, it is best to start an infusion. The main side effects of this treatment are listed in Table 3 but the most significant is apnoea, which may necessitate assisted ventilation.

Heart failure

The presentation of heart failure in infants is with tachypnoea, difficulty in feeding or failure to thrive. The main non-cardiological cause of tachypnoea is lower respiratory tract disorders. Less frequent causes are cerebral abnormalities, acidosis from renal failure and metabolic disorders. Infants in heart failure are tachypnoeic (respiratory rate > 60/min at rest) with intercostal and subcostal recession and have a tachycardia (heart rate > 180/min). They may feed poorly because they become breathless. Sweating is often seen from increased sympathetic activity to compensate for the reduced peripheral blood flow and from their high metabolic rate. On auscultation, there may be a gallop rhythm but this can be difficult to identify with such a rapid heart beat. This gallop rhythm is either an accentuated third heart sound or a combination of the third and fourth heart sounds. A soft third heart sound is often heard in normal infants. Crepitations and wheezing from pulmonary venous congestion are a late manifestation but may also be caused by a chest infection. The liver is enlarged and is palpable more than 2 centimetres below the right costal margin. Peripheral oedema is unusual. Infants with acute heart failure and lower respiratory tract infections have many features in common. The most helpful in distinguishing between them are the presence of hepatomegaly, inappropriate weight gain from fluid retention and cardiomegaly on the chest radiograph in infants in heart failure. The infected child may be febrile and toxic. Both may be present as chest infections are common in infants with heart failure.

Causes

The lesions which may cause heart failure are listed in Table 4. The earlier in life these infants present, the more serious the underlying

212

Table 4   Causes of heart failure in neonates and infants

Obstructive left-sided lesions
   Coarctation of the aorta or interrupted aortic arch
   Critical aortic stenosis
   Hypoplastic left heart syndrome

Large left-to-right shunts

Myocardial disease
   Myocarditis
   Myocardial ischaemia in the neonate

Arrhythmias
   Paroxysmal supraventricular tachycardia

lesion is likely to be. In the first week of life heart failure is usually caused by the hypoplastic left heart syndrome, coarctation of the aorta or complex anomalies. It may also be seen in children with normal hearts who have fluid overload, severe anaemia or in paroxysmal supraventricular tachycardia.

In the hypoplastic left heart syndrome the left ventricle is poorly developed with hypoplasia or atresia of the mitral valve, aortic valve and arch of the aorta. The baby may appear normal at birth, when blood passing through the ductus arteriosus by-passes the obstruction. Within the first few days, as the ductus closes, the baby becomes tachypnoeic and cyanosed with poor peripheral pulses. They have a low cardiac output and are shocked and may initially be thought to be septicaemic. Echocardiography will usually confirm the diagnosis if the baby survives long enough for this to be performed. It is the commonest cause of death from congenital heart disease in the first week of life.

Babies with coarctation of the aorta or an interrupted aortic arch who present in heart failure early in life have severe aortic narrowing. Initially blood flows to the descending aorta via the ductus arteriosus but when it closes they develop heart failure and there is reduced blood flow to the abdomen, kidneys and lower limbs. The femoral pulses become weak or absent and the blood pressure in the arms is at least 20 mmHg higher than in the legs. Infusion of prostaglandin E_1 will be temporarily beneficial by keeping the ductus open prior to surgery.

Preterm infants, especially those with respiratory distress

syndrome may develop heart failure from a patent ductus arteriosus (PDA). This usually occurs towards the end of the first week of life. Clinical features are tachypnoea, a systolic ejection murmur over the pulmonary area and bounding pulses. The chest radiograph may show cardiomegaly and pulmonary plethora. The size of the shunt can be gauged by echocardiography by comparing the diameter of the left atrium to the aortic root. A ratio greater than 1.2 : 1 suggests that the shunt is significant. Many babies will respond to fluid restriction. The arterial oxygen tension is maintained as high as possible without running the risk of retrolental fibroplasia, and the haematocrit is kept high. Frusemide is sometimes given but digoxin appears to be of little or no benefit. Naturally circulating prostaglandins keep the ductus patent and indomethacin, a prostaglandin synthetase inhibitor, has been found to close the ductus in 50 to 75% of cases. If the ductus is preventing the baby from being weaned from artificial ventilation or is causing significant symptoms, and the baby does not have renal insufficiency, oral indomethacin ($0.2\,\mathrm{mg\,kg}^{-1}$ $(8\,\mathrm{h})^{-1}$ three times if necessary) may be given. It seems to be more successful the earlier it is given. If these measures fail, the ductus may need to be ligated surgically.

Investigations

In heart failure cardiomegaly (a transverse cardiothoracic ratio of 60% or more in the first year of life) is usually present on the chest radiograph. The pulmonary vascular markings are often increased (Figure 2) but this may not be evident initially. The ECG may show a range of abnormalities depending on the underlying abnormality.

Management

Rapid and adequate use of diuretics is the most important therapeutic measure. For rapid diuresis in the sick infant frusemide can be given via the intravenous or intramuscular route. The oral route can be used as soon as the baby improves. Potassium loss can be avoided by giving the frusemide with potassium chloride or spironolactone. If it is decided to digitalize the baby, digoxin (Lanoxin) can be given intramuscularly in the sick baby, but should otherwise be given orally. One of the many regimens for digitalization is shown in Table 5. The differences between therapeutic and toxic dosage is small. The

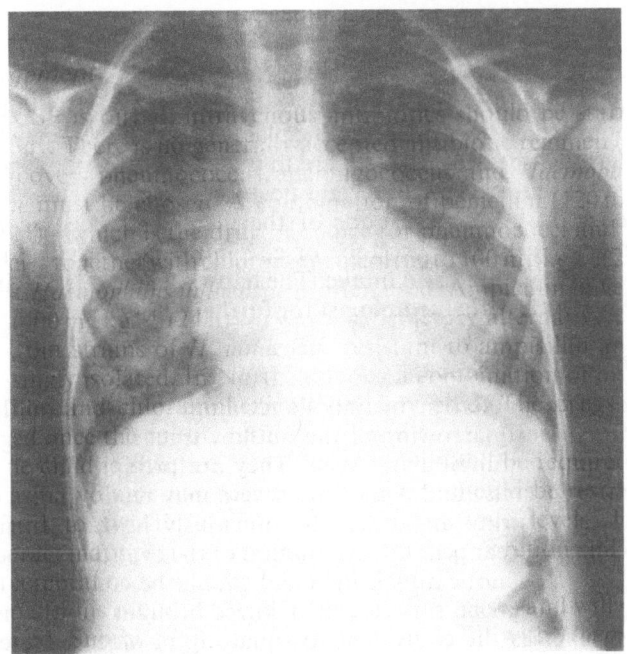

Figure 2 *Chest radiograph of a child in heart failure showing increased pulmonary vasculature and cardiomegaly*

Table 5 Drugs in heart failure

Frusemide i.v., i.m. or p.o. 1 mg/kg given b.d. This dose may be doubled.
Spironolactone p.o. 1.5–3.0 mg kg^{-1} (24 h)$^{-1}$, given b.d. or tds.
Potassium chloride 2 mmol kg^{-1} (24 h)$^{-1}$
Digoxin: Dosage scheme for digitalization using Lanoxin (Burroughs & Wellcome). (After Jordan and Scott, 1981).

Age of patient	Total digitalizing dose given over 24 hours		Maintenance dose/24 hours	
	Oral	Intramuscular	Oral	Intramuscular
Premature or less than 1 month	0.04 mg/kg	0.03 mg/kg	0.010 mg/kg	0.010 mg/kg
1 month to 2 years	0.06 mg/kg	0.04 mg/kg	0.020 mg/kg	0.015 mg/kg
2 years to 10 years	0.04 mg/kg	0.03 mg/kg	0.010 mg/kg	0.010 mg/kg

After the age of 10 adult doses may be used.
The digitalizing dose should be given in three doses. Half the total digitalizing dose is given immediately, then a quarter of the total dose after 8 hours and the remaining quarter of the total dose after a further 8 hours.
The maintenance dose should be given in two divided doses at 12-hourly intervals.

only early clinical features of toxicity in the newborn are vomiting and poor feeding. Bradycardia, supraventricular arrhythmias and heart block may develop later. The plasma digoxin level may be high.

Other therapeutic measures are to nurse the baby in oxygen (30% is usually sufficient) in an upright position either in a chair for older babies or by tilting the floor of the incubator. Feeding may be possible via a nasogastric tube or else intravenous fluids are given with a reduced total fluid intake. The baby must be referred immediately to a paediatric cardiologist for further assessment.

Cyanotic attacks

These are characteristic of Fallot's tetralogy and are thought to be associated with narrowing of the outflow tract from the right ventricle due to infundibular spasm. They are precipitated by crying, feeding or exercise and if they are severe may result in loss of consciousness. During an attack the previously heard murmur may disappear and reappear on termination of the cyanotic episode.

During a cyanotic attack the child should be comforted to calm him. Infants can be sat with their knees brought up against their chests which is the equivalent to squatting in older children. One hundred per cent oxygen should be given via a face mask. Drugs may be given to terminate a prolonged attack, either morphine (0.2 mg/kg) or propranolol (0.1 mg/kg slowly i.v.). Acidosis will usually resolve spontaneously but may need correction if it does not. Digoxin is contraindicated as it increases myocardial contractility and may make the outflow obstruction worse. Cyanotic attacks are an indication for surgical intervention.

Paroxysmal supraventricular tachycardia

This is the commonest arrhythmia in infancy and childhood (Figure 3). It may be recurrent. The tachycardia, at a rate of 200–300/min,

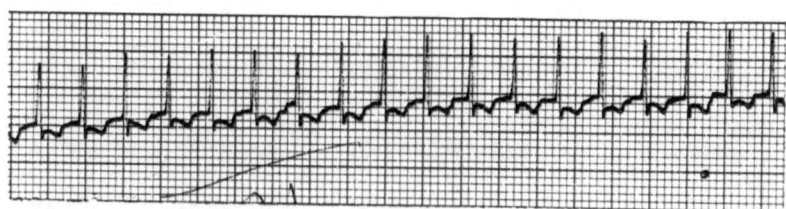

Figure 3   ECG showing supraventricular tachycardia

starts abruptly and may last only minutes, when there are usually few symptoms or up to 24 hours or more, when the child may develop heart failure and become very ill. Older children may describe palpitations accompanied sometimes by dizziness, faintness and abdominal pain. Infants become pale, tachypnoeic and may sweat. Polyuria after termination of an attack is characteristic and may be a clue to the diagnosis. Paroxysmal supraventricular tachycardia may be detected *in utero*.

These tachycardias are mostly thought to be re-entry tachycardias from accessory conducting pathways whilst a few are due to enhanced atrial or atrioventricular node automaticity. Apart from those infants with underlying congenital heart disease and the Wolff–Parkinson-White syndrome the ECG between attacks is normal. It may be possible to demonstrate runs of tachycardia on a 24-hour ECG. Three-quarters of the children have a normal heart, whilst a quarter have underlying congenital heart disease. It may accompany myocarditis, which is usually viral.

Short episodes are well tolerated but with longer attacks infants and neonates are particularly liable to develop heart failure. Vagal stimulation by carotid sinus massage or eyeball pressure may terminate some attacks. If this is ineffective drugs or direct current shock can be used. Intravenous injection of either verapamil (0.05–0.2 mg/kg), disopyramide (2 mg/kg over 5 minutes, then $0.4\,\text{mg}\,\text{kg}^{-1}\,\text{h}^{-1}$) or propranolol (0.1–0.2 mg/kg) can be used. Only one drug should be given at a time. Digoxin can be given intramuscularly and will usually terminate the attack but has the disadvantage that it takes some time to work and makes the subsequent use of direct current shock more hazardous. Diuretics can be added if the infant is in heart failure. In the severely ill patient a synchronized direct current shock (1 J/kg), given under a general anaesthetic or intravenous diazepam, will usually restore sinus rhythm. For the suppression of further attacks, digoxin is the drug of choice but should this be unsuccessful propranolol or disopyramide can be added.

References

Jones, R.S., Baumer, H., Joseph, M.C., and Shinebourne, E.A. (1976). *Arch. Dis. Child.*, **51**, 667

Further reading

Jordan, S.C. and Scott, O. (1981). *Heart Disease in Paediatrics.* Butterworths, London.

Shinebourne, E.A. and Anderson, R.H. (1980). *Current Paediatric Cardiology.* Oxford University Press, Oxford.

Appendix

The following is a guide to the interpretation of the ECG in children. It is useful in the diagnosis of congenital heart disease when considered in conjunction with the findings on clinical examination, the chest radiograph and blood gas results. A serious or lethal cardiac malformation may exist with a normal ECG. In children the ECG must include V_4R.

ECG analysis

(1) Rate and rhythm

Infants have a fast heart rate, and the normal values at different ages are shown in Table 1.

Table 1   Heart rate at different ages

	Heart rate	
Age	Mean	Range
0–24 hours	145	80–200
1–7 days	133	100–175
8–30 days	163	115–190
1–3 months	154	115–205
3–6 months	140	115–205
6–12 months	140	115–175
1–3 years	126	100–190
3–5 years	98	55–145
5–8 years	96	70–145

(2) Atrial hypertrophy
Atrial hypertrophy is present if the P wave in lead II is greater than 0.28 mV at any age.

(3) Abnormalities of conduction
The normal P–R interval is:
0.07–0.12 s if <1 year
0.09–0.16 s if >1 year

(4) Mean frontal QRS axis
Method: Consider leads I and aVF
Count the number of squares of the QRS forces above the line as +ve and below as −ve.
Take the sum of the R (+ve) and S (−ve) wave in I and aVF i.e. height of R wave−height of S wave.
Plot an appropriate axis.
Extend two perpendicular lines and draw a line through the point of intersection to obtain the mean frontal QRS axis (Figure 1).
Normal values for the mean frontal QRS axis are shown in Table 2.

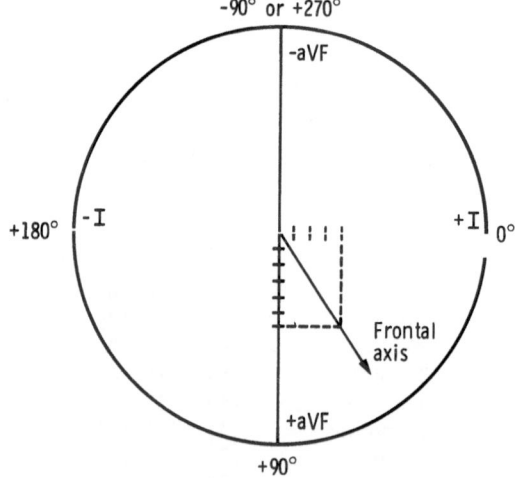

Figure 1 *Orientation of leads I and aVF in the frontal plane, showing an example of how the mean frontal QRS axis is calculated*

Table 2 Normal frontal QRS axis

	Mean	*Range*
0–24 hours	135	60–180
1–7 days	125	60–180
8–30 days	110	0–180
1–3 months	80	20–120
3–6 months	65	40–100
6–12 months	65	20–120
1–3 years	55	0–120
3–5 years	60	0–80
5–8 years	65	−20–100

The mean frontal QRS axis is best stated in degrees. The term 'superior axis deviation' is preferable to 'left axis deviation' and it is present if the QRS forces in aVF are dominantly negative. Its presence is strongly suggestive of congenital heart disease, especially endocardial cushion defect or a large ventriculoseptal defect. In a cyanosed infant it may indicate a univentricular heart with or without an absent right atrioventricular connexion (tricuspid atresia).

Criteria for ventricular hypertrophy

Hypertrophy is assessed from the R and S voltages and T wave patterns on the chest leads.

Right ventricular hypertrophy

Tall R in V_4R > 20 mV under 1 week
                      > 15 mV 1 week to 3 months
                      > 10 mV over 1 year
Deep S in V_6 > 15 mV under 1 week
                      > 10 mV 1 week to 3 months
                      > 5 mV over 1 year
Upright T in V_4R, V_1 after 1 week of age

Left ventricular hypertrophy

Tall R in V_6 > 12 mV under 1 week
                      > 20 mV 1 week to 3 months
                      > 25 mV over 1 year

Deep S in $V_4R > 20\,mV$ under 1 week
　　　　　 $> 15\,mV$ 1 week to 1 month
　　　　　 $> 20\,mV$ over 1 month
Inverted T in V_5V_6
Right or left ventricular hypertrophy should be diagnosed only if both V_4R and V_6 are abnormal.

Biventricular hypertrophy

R + S waves in V_3 and V_4 exceed 70 mV.

CHAPTER 14

Accidents and poisoning

It is estimated that in England and Wales over 2 million children between 1 and 14 years old attend hospital each year following accidents. This is as many as 1 in every 5 children. At all ages boys have more accidents than girls. Most of the injuries will be minor but many are more serious and some children are left with permanent handicaps. Accidents remain the commonest cause of death in children over 1 year old. Although the number of deaths has been declining, in 1979, in England and Wales, 925 children between 1 and 14 years died from accidents, accounting for 30% of all deaths in this age group. Road traffic accidents constitute the commonest cause followed by drowning and burns (Table 1).

The nature of an accident is related to a child's age and stage of development. Toddlers are constantly exploring and are unaware of the consequences of their actions. They are often indoors and are frequently involved in injuries from scalds and burns, falls, drowning and accidental poisoning. Young children who are still inexperienced with traffic are particularly at risk from motor accidents. Older children are at risk both as pedestrians and cyclists and are also involved in falls from trees and roofs. The home and social circumstances influence childhood accidents. The preventative measures taken to reduce risk factors and the level of supervision vary considerably between families. There also tend to be more accidents in homes with a high level of stress. Some children or families seem particularly accident-prone and this may be a reflection both of

Table 1   Causes of accidental death in childhood in 1979 in England and Wales, expressed as percentages. (Source—Office of Population Censuses and Surveys)

Accident	Age group		
	1-4 y	*5-9 y*	*10-14 y*
Motor traffic accidents	38.4	61.9	58.6
collision with pedestrian	(29.8)	(50.8)	(29.5)
collision with cyclist	(0.4)	(4.8)	(22.3)
Drowning, submersion, suffocation	19.8	17.2	10.7
Fires and flames	16.7	6.0	6.0
Falls	6.6	3.9	4.5
Others	18.6	10.9	20.2
Number of deaths	258	331	336

their personalities and the level of stress in the household. With these families care should not be confined to the individual injuries but should include a more comprehensive assessment of the family situation involving the health visitor and social worker.

Head injury

Head injuries, especially from road traffic accidents or falls, are a common cause of death, permanent handicap and seizures. There are two main groups of children seen in the accident and emergency department: those who have been subjected to severe trauma and have a reduced level of consciousness and clearly require medical attention, and the much more sizeable group who have recovered fully by the time they are seen. It is in this latter group that sometimes a difficult decision has to be made whether the child needs to be admitted to hospital for a period of observation or can be sent home.

Admission to hospital

It is best, in general, to admit any child where the history suggests a severe blow and any child who has lost consciousness, even momentarily. The absence of a skull fracture should not be regarded as the deciding factor as there may be extensive brain damage without a fracture. Any child who has sustained a blow severe enough to

224

fracture the skull should be admitted, especially if the fracture crosses the groove of the middle meningeal artery. A child must always be admitted if there is leakage of blood or CSF from the nose, bilateral periorbital haematomas, conjunctival haemorrhage without a clearly defined limit or a haematoma over the mastoid as any of these may indicate a basal skull fracture. It is not uncommon for young children to vomit and briefly become pale following trauma to the head but any child who vomits persistently, remains or becomes increasingly drowsy or unwell should be admitted. Whenever child abuse is suspected admission to hospital is indicated for further evaluation.

Cerebral oedema

The most frequent complication is cerebral oedema. It is more common in children as their skulls are softer and more easily distorted than adults. In an adult, the force of the impact is taken by the skull, whereas in a child the skull distorts and the impact is transmitted to the brain causing severe stresses and pressure waves. The resulting damage and cerebral oedema may give rise to loss of consciousness, pallor and vomiting which may last from hours to several days.

Intracranial haemorrhage

Intracranial haemorrhage, either extradural or subdural, occurs less often. Extradural haemorrhage usually results from damage to the middle meningeal artery. There is often but not always an underlying skull fracture. It is of rapid onset, unilateral, and the lucid interval immediately after the blow seen in adults is unusual in children. Subdural haematomas are mainly seen in infants. In many cases there is no skull fracture. They are mostly bilateral, and often cause seizures. The regular observations made in hospital on patients with head injuries are intended to detect an intracranial haemorrhage or a sudden rise in cerebral oedema. These events may be indicated by a fall in the level of consciousness, a falling pulse rate, a rising blood pressure and changes in the size and reactivity of the pupils. A unilaterally dilated and unreactive pupil suggests temporal lobe herniation from a unilateral lesion. A CT scan will usually show the site and extent of an intracranial haemorrhage. If the patient's condition does not allow time for this to be performed and an intracranial bleed is suspected, three exploratory burr holes one in the frontal, one parietal and one temporal are made on each side of the skull to remove any blood clot and stop further bleeding.

Burns and scalds

The consequences of an extensive burn may be severe, including scarring, deformity, disability and psychological upset for both the child and his family. Scalds are especially common in young children. The best immediate treatment of burns and scalds is not always appreciated in the home and folk remedies often prevail. Immediately after a scald, the clothes over which hot fluid has spilt should be removed. Small scalds and burns can be cooled under cold running water until the pain is relieved. Burns or scalds should be covered only with a clean sheet or towel before coming to hospital.

In the accident and emergency department, as with any seriously injured child, an adequate airway must be ensured and then anxiety and pain relieved and the extent of the burn assessed (Table 2). If

Table 2   Estimate of the percentage of the body area of a burn

	Percentage of whole child			
	Newborn	3 years	6 years	> 12 years
Head	18	15	12	6
Trunk	40	40	40	38
Arms	16	14	16	18
Legs	26	29	32	38

The surface area of the patient's palm with the fingers closed is approximately 1%. Perineum is 1"„. The hand is a quarter of the upper limb. The foot is one sixth of the lower limb, from the ankle to the knee two-sixth of the lower limb and the leg above the knee three-sixths.

more than 10% of the surface area is involved, excluding the surrounding erythema, intravenous fluids are necessary to counteract the loss of plasma volume and prevent shock from hypovolaemia. In Britain the standard regimen (Muir and Barclay, 1974) is to give colloid, either plasma, plasma protein fraction or Haemaccel, and to calculate the fluid given in the first 4 hours from the time of the accident according to the formula:

colloid in ml = 0.5 × total surface area of burnt skin (in %)
× weight in kg.

Crystalloids like Ringer's lactate are preferred in many other countries, as it is thought that most of the fluid loss is from fluid shifting from the intravascular to the extravascular compartment rather than loss from the burn itself and that giving large volumes of colloid makes the affected areas more oedematous. Subsequent fluid therapy is regulated according to the clinical response, urine output and the serum and urine electrolytes and osmolality. Initially there is haemoconcentration, but the haematocrit then falls and will also need to be monitored. If analgesia is required, it can be given via the intravenous infusion (e.g. morphine 0.1–0.2 mg/kg). Tetanus toxoid booster should be given.

Whilst the degree of systemic illness is determined by the extent of the body area involved, the eventual outcome of a particular burn is determined by the depth of tissue damage. This can be difficult to assess accurately but if sensation is present to pinprick the burn is of partial thickness and will heal spontaneously. If there is analgesia, skin grafting will probably be needed.

Admission to hospital is advisable for all young children with anything but the most minor burns. All children with more than 7% of the skin involved must be admitted, or if the burn involves the eye, face and neck, hands or perineum unless they are extremely minor. Children who have been in a smoke-filled room must be admitted for 24 hours observation even if they do not have any respiratory symptoms at the time as these may develop subsequently. Admission will be required if child abuse is suspected. The severely burned child must be referred immediately to a specialist burns unit.

The scalded skin syndrome

The scalded skin syndrome (Figure 1) in children is not due to heat injury, in spite of the name, but to staphylococcal infection. It is also called toxic epidermal necrolysis (Ritter's disease in neonates, Lyell's disease in children). There is widespread erythema of the skin, which becomes tender, and the skin is denuded by the slightest pressure (Nikolsky's sign). The epidermal cleavage is due to a toxin of *Staphylococcus aureus* (mostly phage type 71). Treatment is with antibiotics against the staphylococcus. Flucloxacillin can be used, and is initially given intravenously. The skin must be handled very gently and precautions taken to avoid infection and hypothermia. In adults this syndrome may be caused by drugs but this is very rare in children.

227

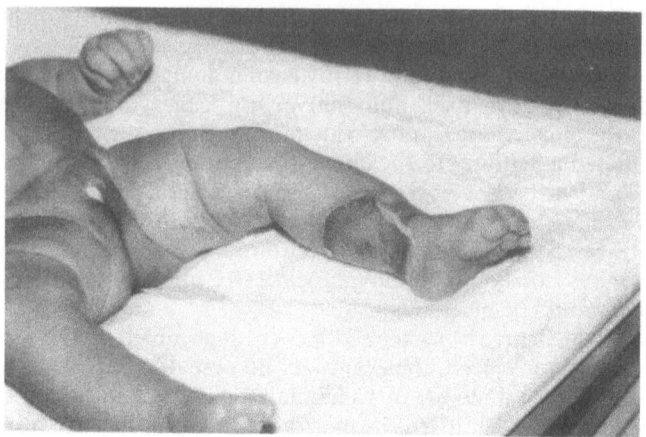

Figure 1   *An infant with the scalded skin syndrome*

Bullous impetigo is a more localized form of the scalded skin syndrome.

Poisoning

Poisoning in children is extremely common and constitutes over a fifth of all paediatric medical admissions. Fortunately most cases are mild with relatively few children having any symptoms at all. Fatalities are rare. In England and Wales about 20 children die each year from poisoning. In 1979 only 5 children died from the ingestion of medicines.

Most cases of poisoning involve overdoses of medicines (53%), but ingestion of household products (38%) and berries, seeds and fungi (6%) are also common. The vast majority of cases are accidental involving toddlers between one and four years old. In most of the cases only small quantities are ingested, and often a child is found playing with tablets and it is not clear if any have been taken at all. In older children, particularly adolescents, drug overdose may be deliberate. Occasionally drugs may be given by parents as a form of child abuse. Overdosage may be iatrogenic either from an incorrect dose, the drug may be inappropriate for children (e.g. phenoxylate (Lomotil)) or when an inadvisable combination of drug is used (e.g.

228

prochlorperazine (Stemetil) and metaclopramide (Maxolon)) (Figure 2).

The availability of drugs and harmful substances in the home is an important factor in the incidence of accidents. It is often when visiting the homes of grandparents or people without children that toddlers find drugs in easily accessible places. Poisonous substances decanted into containers which normally hold food or drinks are particularly dangerous. Psychosocial factors also appear important and an increased number of accidents including poisoning may reflect a parti-

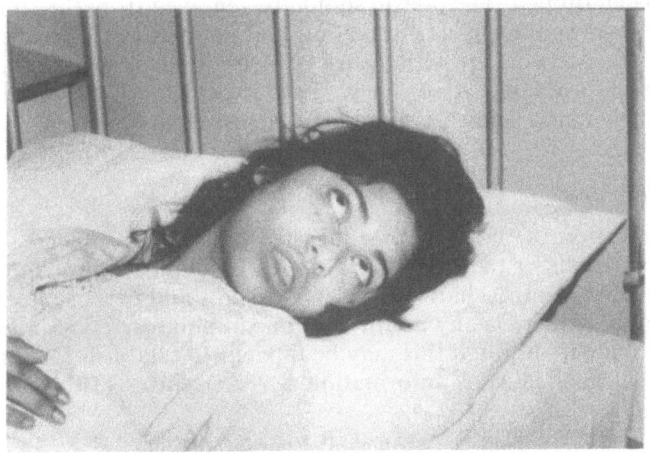

Figure 2 *Oculogyric crisis from a combination of prochlorperazine (Stemetil) and metoclopramide (Maxolon)*

cularly active or impulsive child, an adverse home environment or a high level of family stress.

Attempts to prevent accidental poisoning have been made by educational campaigns directed at parents and the general public. Parents are encouraged to lock medicines in cupboards especially designed so that children cannot open them. This has not proved particularly successful, but more success has been achieved by supplying medicines in containers which children find difficult to open. Since 1977 aspirin and paracetamol for both children and adults have had to be dispensed in child resistant containers. The number of hospital admissions for analgesic poisoning in children under 5 years in 1978 was only a quarter of the number for 1974. Other factors which may possibly have contributed to this decrease is that the number of paediatric tablets dispensed is limited to 25 and the publicity surrounding the introduction of these changes may have increased public awareness.

Management

The management follows a similar pattern whatever the agent ingested. The agent must be identified and the maximum possible dose taken determined. The poison should be removed from the stomach unless contraindicated. Observation and support are the most important aspects of care with the use of an antidote or specific therapy if they are available. Assessment of the social situation surrounding the incident and aftercare should not be forgotten.

Identification

Identification of the substance ingested is usually provided by the child's parents or they may bring some of the tablets or a container with them. Identity charts of tablets or plants and berries may be of assistance if there is any doubt. The maximum dose taken needs to be estimated, although this may be difficult to establish for certain. The National Poisons Information Service centres (Table 3) may

Table 3   National Poisons Information Service centres in Britain

Belfast	0232-30503
Cardiff	0222-492233
Edinburgh	031-229-2477
London	01-407-7600
Other centres	
Leeds	0532-32799
Manchester	061-740-2254

provide information and can be especially helpful in providing details of the constituents and toxicity of the many different household products which are ingested. The information given is not specific for children and does not provide advice on how to manage a particular patient.

Removal of the poison

The effects of poisoning can be prevented or reduced if the ingested poison can be removed from the stomach before absorption takes place. In children this is best achieved by inducing vomiting with syrup of ipecacuanha (Table 4). If vomiting is not induced in 20 minutes, the dose should be repeated. The child will vomit in well over 90% of cases and this seems to include overdoses of antiemetics.

Vomiting is quicker, kinder and more effective in removing ingested toxic contents than gastric lavage. It is contraindicated if

Table 4   Induction of emesis in a child

Method
Syrup of ipecacuanha, 15 ml taken with a glass of water or fruit juice

Indications
Ingestion of a potentially toxic dose of poison
Less than 6 hours since ingestion, or within 12–24 h for salicylates, anticholinergic drugs like tricyclic antidepressants, diphenoxylate (Lomotil), iron

Contraindications
Impaired level of consciousness
Poisoning from corrosives
Poisoning from petroleum distillates

consciousness is impaired, after ingestion of corrosives as it may extend the area of ulceration or cause perforation and after the ingestion of petroleum distillates like paraffin or turpentine as they may be inhaled and result in lipoid pneumonia.

Gastric lavage is rarely necessary in children. It is required if the child is unconscious, but only after they have been intubated with a cuffed endotracheal tube. It is also used for some specific ingestions, for example, paraquat, and will enable an antidote to be left in the stomach. It is contraindicated with corrosives or petroleum distillates.

Activated charcoal

Activated charcoal has an enormous adsorptive surface area and will adsorb a wide range of drugs and chemicals. Although its capability for adsorption *in vitro* is undeniable its efficacy *in vivo* is difficult to demonstrate. One problem is that it is not very palatable though this has been somewhat improved by the introduction of a finely ground effervescent charcoal (Medicoal) (0.5-1 g/kg with water). Its other major limitation is that it needs to be given in doses of 5 to 10 times the estimated weight of poison to achieve a significant reduction in drug adsorption; a 10 g dose of activated charcoal might adsorb up to forty 25 mg amitriphyline tablets but only two 500 mg paracetamol tablets. As it will bind the syrup of ipecacuanha, it should only be given after emesis has been induced. It is most likely to be helpful when small quantities of a poison produce a large effect e.g. tricyclic antidepressants or for delayed release drugs such as some theophylline preparations.

Observation and supportive care

Any child who has taken a potentially toxic agent will need to be kept under observation and this usually necessitates admission to hospital. The decision whether or not to admit the child will be influenced not only by the toxicity of the agent but also by the social circumstances. Factors to consider are whether or not the child can be reliably observed at home, the distance from the hospital and if transport is readily available. Admission to hospital will always be required for any child with symptoms.

Any child admitted needs to be closely monitored bearing in mind the particular effects of the poison he has taken. In the severely affected child supportive therapy may be required for respiratory depression, shock, cardiac arrhythmias or temperature instability.

Specific therapy or antidotes are only applicable to a small number of poisons and these are discussed in the appropriate sections.

Aftercare

The circumstances surrounding any poisoning incident need careful assessment. Contact with health visitors or social workers is often helpful to provide additional information about the family and to provide advice and support after discharge. In cases of deliberate overdose in older children psychiatric help will be needed.

Salicylates

Salicylate ingestion is usually of junior aspirin. Other preparations are adult aspirin and occasionally oil of wintergreen (methyl salicylate) which has an extremely high concentration of salicylate. For moderately severe poisoning more than 240 mg/kg needs to be ingested, whilst more than 450 mg/kg may be lethal (Done, 1960).

The early signs of severe salicylate poisoning (Table 5) are nausea,

Table 5   Clinical features of salicylate poisoning

Nausea, vomiting, epigastric pain, hyperpyrexia and sweating
Hyperventilation, pulmonary oedema
Tinnitus, deafness, irritability, tremor, drowsiness, coma
Dehydration, hypokalaemia
Respiratory alkalosis rapidly followed by metabolic acidosis
Hypo- or hyperglycaemia, hypoprothrombinaemia.

vomiting, tinnitus, hyperpyrexia and sweating. The stage of hyperventilation with a respiratory alkalosis is brief or absent in children, who quickly develop a metabolic acidosis. This early onset of acidosis means less salicylate is excreted and also the salicylate penetrates tissues more readily and in particular enhances central nervous system toxicity. Dehydration is an early feature, and there may be hypo- or hyperglycaemia. Coma is unusual unless the overdose is very severe.

Following the ingestion of a small dose of aspirin, the peak serum level is reached in about an hour, but with a large dose the peak may be only at 4-6 hours, and may even continue to rise for up to 24 hours as the tablets adhere to each other and dissolve only slowly as gastric emptying is delayed. Emesis should be induced up to 24 hours after ingestion, and the child admitted to hospital. A blood salicylate level is helpful as symptoms may be slow in developing. Salicylates can readily be detected in the urine with a Phenistix, which turns brownish-purple, and a negative result more than an hour after ingestion suggests that an insignificant amount was taken.

The severity of the overdose can be assessed using a nomogram (Figure 3). If the initial salicylate level is greater than 500 mg/l or if the child has symptoms, an intravenous infusion should be started and the urea, electrolytes, blood glucose, prothrombin time and

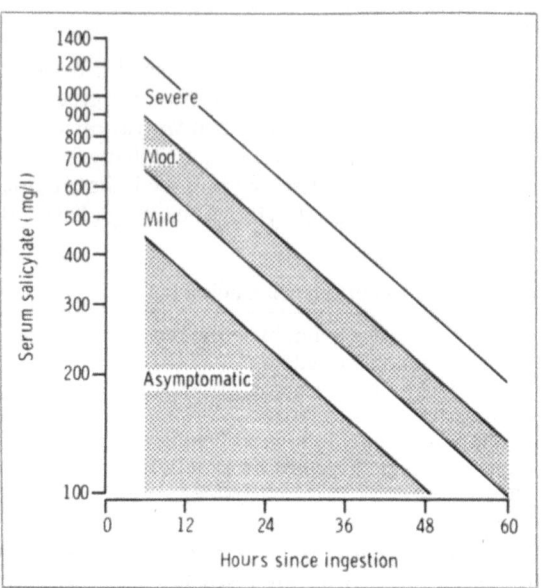

Figure 3 *Nomogram relating serum salicylate to severity of intoxication following acute ingestion of aspirin. The nomogram starts at 6 hours to ensure a peak level. It can be used earlier, but a further level is needed to establish that it is not increasing. Adapted with permission from Done, 1960*

blood gases need to be monitored. Vitamin K is given for the hypo-prothrombinaemia. It is important to prevent dehydration and the deleterious effects of a marked metabolic acidosis can be avoided by correcting it with sodium bicarbonate, taking care to avoid hypo-kalaemia. In children it tends to be difficult to get the urine sufficiently alkaline (pH > 7.5) to achieve a forced alkaline diuresis without overloading the circulation with sodium and water. For the very severe case, salicylate may be removed by dialysis.

Paracetamol

Paracetamol (acetaminophen) is used extensively as an antipyretic and analgesic. Accidental ingestion is not uncommon but it is extremely rare for a child to ingest sufficient (more than 150 mg/kg) to have any serious consequences.

The clinical features of paracetamol overdose are listed in Table 6.

Table 6   Clinical features of severe paracetamol overdose

1st day	Anorexia, nausea, vomiting
1st–2nd day	Abdominal pain
	Abnormal liver function tests (after 12–36 h):
	Bilirubin, Aspartate aminotransferase
	Prothrombin time
2nd–7th day	Hepatic failure
	Also acute renal failure, cardiac arrhythmias

When managing a patient who has taken an overdose of paracetamol it is important to remember that there is a delay of up to a day before the onset of symptoms from the most serious consequence, hepatic failure. Other serious problems are acute renal failure and cardiac arrythmias. Hypoglycaemia, temperature instability and a metabolic acidosis may also be seen.

Emesis should be induced. A plasma paracetamol level will tell whether hepatic toxicity is likely (Figure 4). If the initial level is taken within four hours, a second sample will need to be taken more than

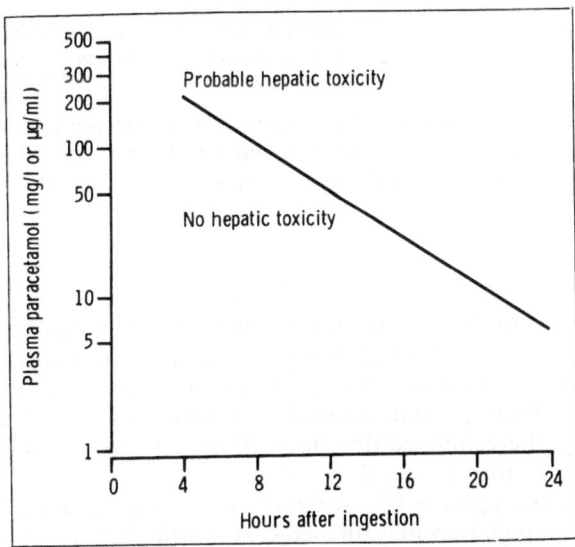

Figure 4 *Nomogram relating the dose of paracetamol ingested and the like-lihood of hepatic toxicity. Reproduction with permission from Rumack and Matthews, 1975*

4 hours after ingestion to ensure that the maximum level has been reached. Some patients with serum paracetamol levels above the line will still have only minimal liver damage. In patients at risk of hepatic failure, methionine or *N*-acetyl-cysteine will reduce the severity of liver necrosis by increasing the available glutathione. A small fraction of paracetamol is normally metabolized by a mixed function oxidase enzyme (cytochrome P450) to a reactive metabolite which normally complexes with glutathione. In paracetamol overdosage there is insufficient glutathione to form complexes with the toxic metabolite. Acetyl cysteine (Mucomyst) which is used in the treatment of cystic fibrosis can be given (Table 7). The oral solution tastes unpleasant

Table 7   Dosage of *N*-acetyl-cysteine and methionine for severe paracetamol overdose (After Vale and Meredith 1981)

N-Acetyl-cysteine	i.v.	150 mg/kg over 15 min, then 50 mg/kg in next 4 h then 100 mg/kg over next 16 h
	oral	140 mg/kg, then 70 mg/kg every 4 hours Dilute 20% solution to a 5% solution
Methionine	p.o.	Adult dose is 2.5 g start, then 2.5 g every 4 hours for further 3 doses

and vomiting is common. In Britain, acetyl cysteine has been used intravenously and methionine, given orally, has also been used. Neither preparation is effective if given more than 10 hours after ingestion.

Iron

Iron tablets prescribed for pregnant mothers will often be found in a toddler's home. They are now dispensed in bubble packets which may have contributed to the reduced incidence of severe iron poisoning. Only a small number of tablets may produce serious poisoning. It is estimated that three of the standard ferrous sulphate tablets per kg may be lethal.

Three clinical phases following severe iron ingestion are described (Table 8) though they may all merge. A fourth phase is the long term complications from scarring of the stomach.

The severity is assessed from the history, whether there are any symptoms and the serum iron. A serum iron above 90 µmol/l (500 µg/

Table 8   Clinical features of severe iron overdosage

Phase	Clinical features
Immediate from local toxicity	Vomiting, diarrhoea, abdominal pain, haematemesis and melaena. Dehydration
Latent interval (6-16 hours)	Improvement
Systemic toxicity (12-24 hours)	Encephalopathy-seizures, coma Circulatory collapse
Late complications	Gastrointestinal strictures from scarring

100 ml) suggests serious iron poisoning, although the actual level does not correlate well with the severity of intoxication. As iron tablets are radio-opaque, a straight abdominal radiograph can be used to identify the number present in the stomach. Depending on the severity of the overdose the child may be given only ipecac. to induce emesis, or this can be followed by passing a nasogastric tube and irrigating the stomach with 1% sodium bicarbonate and then leaving 5 g in 100 ml of the chelating agent desferioxamine in the stomach. For the severe overdose gastric lavage is often recommended. If the child is symptomatic or has ingested a large amount of iron (more than 40 mg/kg of elemental iron) an intramuscular injection of desferioxamine (500 mg/kg) should be given immediately. If the child is collapsed and the serum iron is very high, the desferioxamine is also given intravenously ($15 \, mg \, kg^{-1} \, h^{-1}$ to maximum dose of $80 \, mg \, kg^{-1} (24 \, h)^{-1}$). The iron can be removed by dialysis if this therapy is ineffective. Supportive management especially of the fluid balance is also important.

Lomotil

Lomotil, which is used as an antidiarrhoeal agent in adults, is a mixture of a narcotic diphenoxylate and atropine. It may result in serious toxicity and death in children.

These drugs delay gastric emptying and reduce intestinal motility so the onset of symptoms may be delayed and there may be relapse during recovery. The dose ingested does not appear to correlate well with the severity of symptoms. Initial symptoms are from the atropine but after about 3 hours the narcotic effects of the diphenoxylate predominate. Mildly affected patients experience primarily the

237

atropinic effects with tachycardia, flushing, urinary retention, restlessness and excitement but the pupils are constricted from the diphenoxylate. In those who are more severely affected this will be followed by drowsiness, respiratory depression or coma.

All children who have ingested Lomotil should be admitted for monitoring of their respirations and level of consciousness. Facilities for ventilatory support must be available. The stomach contents should be removed up to 24 hours after ingestion. Activated charcoal has been recommended, especially as there is prolonged excretion by the enterohepatic circulation. If the child is drowsy or there is respiratory depression naloxone is indicated to reverse these effects. The initial dose is 0.01 mg/kg intravenously, and if there is no response within 2 minutes giving a larger dose of 0.1 mg/kg has been suggested (Moore et al., 1980). As the duration of action of the naloxone (one to four hours) is shorter than that of the diphenoxylate further doses may be required.

Lomotil should never be prescribed for young children. It is ineffective as an antidiarrhoeal agent in young children, and as there is poor correlation between the severity of symptoms and the dose given the toxic dose in children cannot be predicted.

Tricyclic antidepressants

Amitryptyline (Tryptizol) and imipramine (Tofranil) are the standard preparations and are prescribed for adults with depression or for a child's enuresis. These drugs have atropine-like effects, exert cerebral stimulation, respiratory depression and, most dangerous of all, may produce cardiac dysrhythmias (Table 9). Symptoms appear within 30–60 min and are maximal in 4–16 hours.

In the poisoned patient, there is initially a sinus tachycardia, dry mouth, dilated pupils and excitement which may alternate with drowsiness. The tendon reflexes are increased with extensor plantar responses. With more serious overdosage the patient may experience hallucinations, convulsions or coma. Cardiac arrhythmias arise from decreased myocardial contractility and increased conduction time. The arrhythmias include sinus bradycardia, supraventricular and ventricular tachycardias, sinus rhythm with grossly prolonged atrioventricular and intraventricular conduction, ventricular fibrillation and cardiac arrest.

Emesis should be induced. Activated charcoal may be useful as the

Table 9   Clinical features of tricyclic antidepressants

Atropine-like	Dry mouth
	Blurred vision
	Dilated pupils
	Sinus tachycardia
	Urinary retention, paralytic ileus
CNS stimulant	Agitation, twitching
	Hallucinations
	Convulsions
	Coma
Cardiovascular	Bradycardia
system	Ventricular tachycardia and fibrillation
	Asystole
	Hypertension
Respiratory	Respiratory depression
	Apnoea

weight of drug ingested is small and there is enterohepatic recirculation. It is possible to reverse the atropine-like effects with physostigmine, a cholinesterase inhibitor. Although it will improve the level of consciousness its effects are short-acting and it may produce convulsions. If used at all, it is restricted to patients with prolonged coma. Some cardiac arrhythmias may be reversed with correction of any metabolic acidosis but profound bradycardia would require cardiac pacing, although even this may not be successful if the myocardium is severely damaged.

Paraquat

When the weedkiller paraquat is ingested it produces damage to the lungs, liver and kidney but the final outcome is dependent on the severity of the pulmonary fibrosis, which has a delayed onset but is progressive and irreversible. There is no treatment to prevent or ameliorate it. Ingestion of as little as 10 ml of the concentrated form of paraquat (Gramoxone, 20% paraquat), in an adult, may be lethal whilst ingestion of small quantities of the less concentrated granular preparations (Weedol) is likely to be favourable. Gastric lavage is recommended, and to leave a mixture of a 30% suspension of Fuller's earth and magnesium sulphate. If given within 30 minutes of ingestion it may delay further absorption, and it should be repeated 4 hourly.

Alcohol

Severe hypoglycaemia may develop after alcohol ingestion in small children. The degree of hypoglycaemia is unpredictable. It may be possible to prevent the hypoglycaemia by frequent feeds containing glucose or a continuous intravenous infusion of 10% Dextrose. The blood glucose will need to be monitored regularly.

Household products

Household products are often ingested by toddlers either because they are inquisitive or because toxic substances are transferred to containers which usually hold food or drink. It is not uncommon, for instance, for turpentine or white spirit used to clean paint brushes to be transferred to a wide-rimmed container like a jam jar.

Whilst potential toxicity may be high, fortunately so little is usually taken that damage is slight. In contrast corrosives are extremely hazardous, particularly oven cleaners which are 30% caustic soda and dishwashing machine powder which contains caustic salicylates and metasilicates which cause similar lesions to caustic soda ingestion. Ingestion of a concentrated alkali is rapidly followed by deeply penetrating ulceration. This may be seen in the mouth and oesophagus, but the stomach is spared because of the protective effect of gastric acid. These ulcers are extremely painful. Perforation of the oesophagus and respiratory obstruction from laryngeal and glottic oedema have been reported. A late complication is oesophagneal stricture. Emesis or gastric lavage risk further damage and are contraindicated. If the child has lesions in the mouth, and especially retrosternal or epigastric pain, a paediatric thoracic surgeon should be consulted regarding endoscopy. Early endoscopy is generally advised to assess the extent of the lesion so that a rational plan for further management can be made. Steroids to try and reduce the inflammation and stricture formation as well as broad spectrum antibiotics are often recommended.

240

Lead poisoning

In Britain, lead poisoning is rarely seen and only about 100 cases a year of abnormally high lead absorption are recognized. This contrasts with the USA where some 40 000 cases are identified, mostly by screening programmes.

Sources

Children ingest or inhale lead from the environment. Most serious lead poisoning in children is from the ingestion of old lead-based household paint. Children swallow flakes of paint or chew painted surfaces and are at high risk when houses with lead-based paint are renovated and the paint stripped off. Other potential sources are contamination of water or food. Lead-containing water pipes or storage tanks are a potent source of lead in areas with soft and acidic water supplies. Acidic food may be contaminated if it is fermented or stored in old pewter or imperfectly glazed ceramic utensils. Asian families may use surma and other lead-based cosmetics. Lead may be inhaled from burning casings of car batteries. There has recently been concern over the possible detrimental effects of atmospheric lead from exhaust fumes from motor vehicles and industry.

Diagnosis

The diagnosis is based on the history and clinical features and from screening tests. The level of a haem precursor, the free erythrocyte protoporphyrin (FEP), is used for screening. This is not specific for lead, and is increased disproportionately in the presence of iron-deficiency anaemia. The serum lead is used as a guide to the severity of the poisoning, in conjunction with the FEP level, but there is considerable variation in the symptomatology seen at a given lead level. Whenever the diagnosis is suspected, a plain abdominal radiograph should be performed to see if there are any lead-containing objects in the gastrointestinal tract (Figure 5). Radiographs of a knee or wrist may show 'lead lines', dense metaphyseal bands at the growing ends of bones which are seen with chronic ingestion of lead (Figure 6). Late manifestations are anaemia, basophil stippling of neutrophils and the Fanconi syndrome with aminoaciduria, glycosuria and phosphaturia.

241

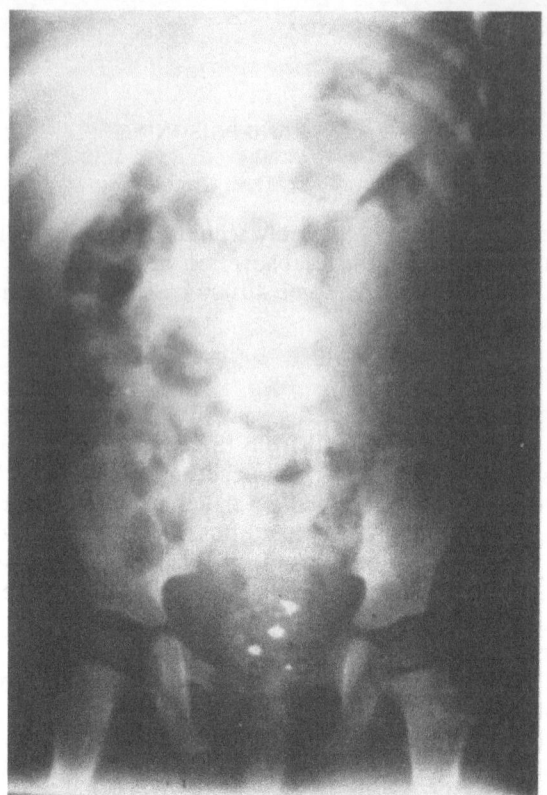

Figure 5 *All children with a raised blood lead should have a plain abdominal radiograph. Flakes of lead-based paint can be seen in this radiograph*

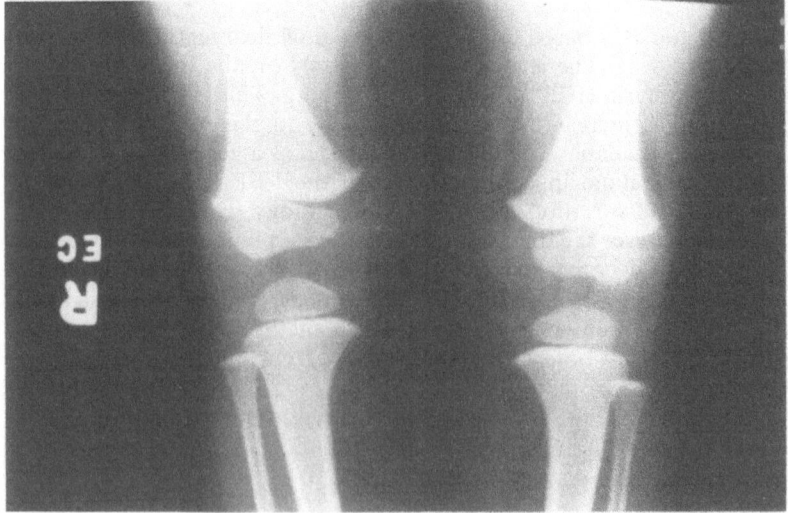

Figure 6 *Lead lines, dense metaphyseal bands at the growing ends of bones from chronic ingestion of lead*

Clinical features

Most children detected by screening programmes are asymptomatic. It has been suggested but not proven that chronically raised blood levels are associated with impaired intellectual performance, behaviour disturbance and minor defects in co-ordination. It might be expected that in children between birth and two years, the period of most rapid neurodevelopment, the brain might be particularly susceptible to toxic insults and there is some evidence that moderate sustained raised blood levels (50–60 µg/100 ml) during early infancy carry a significant risk of subtle neurobehavioural impairment in later childhood. Early symptoms are non-specific, with abdominal pain, constipation and lassitude, whilst severe lead poisoning can result in encephalopathy with irritability, convulsions and coma from an extensive cerebral vasculopathy and cerebral oedema. Raised intracranial pressure with papilloedema may be present. By this stage there is a high incidence of neurological handicap in those who survive.

Management

Priority must be given to removing the source of lead from the child. In spite of this the blood level may continue to rise for some time and the child's condition become progressively more severe. Thereafter, the blood level falls but it may take several months to return to normal. The blood level can be reduced with chelation using penicillamine, calcium-EDTA or dimercaprol (BAL, British Anti-Lewisite) (Table 10). However, they all have potentially serious side-effects, especially the nephrotic syndrome and neutropoenia with penicillamine, and each case needs careful evaluation before therapy is started. These agents will also remove zinc and trace elements which are

Table 10   Drugs used for the chelation of lead

Drugs	Dosage $(mg\,m^{-2}(24\,h)^{-1})$	Route	Contraindications
D-Penicillamine	600	p.o.	Renal disease
Ca-EDTA	1500	i.v. or i.m.	Renal disease
Dimercaprol (BAL)	500	deep i.m.	Liver disease G6PD deficiency

protective of the toxicity of lead. For children with encephalopathy both Ca-EDTA and BAL are given, as well as supportive therapy and management of cerebral oedema. A rebound in the blood lead can be anticipated and can be prevented with penicillamine orally. The management of less severe lead poisoning is controversial, and the regimen suggested in Table 11 is only a guide. Of paramount importance is to check that the source of the lead is removed, and blood levels must be regularly monitored on a long-term basis.

Table 11   Guide to treatment of lead poisoning. (Adapted from Chisholm and Baltrop, 1979 and Baltrop, D. in *Poisoning*, Update Books, 1981)

Serum lead μg/dl (<30 normal)	Additional features	Therapy
30–50	Asymptomatic	Reduce exposure
50–60	Asymptomatic <2 y old–FEP > 300 μg/100 ml >2 y old–FEP > 500 μg/100 ml	Penicillamine
60–80	Asymptomatic	
>80	Asymptomatic or mild symptoms	Ca-EDTA for 7 days (100 mg/m² for last 2 days) ± BAL for 48–72 h
>80	Impending encephalopathy or encephalopathy or very high serum lead	Ca-EDTA + BAL for 5 days

References and further reading

Chambers, T.L. (1981). Child-resistant containers for drugs. *Arch. Dis. Child.*, **56,** 739.

Chisolm, J.J. and Barltrop, D. (1979). Recognition and management of children with increased lead absorption. *Arch. Dis. Child.*, **54,** 249.

Curtis, J.A. and Goel, K.H. (1979). Lomotil poisoning in children. *Arch. Dis. Child.*, **54,** 222.

Done, A.K. (1960). Salicylate intoxication: significance of measurements of salicylate in blood in cases of acute ingestion. *Pediatrics*, **26,** 800.

Done, A.K. (1978). Aspirin overdosage: incidence, diagnosis and management. *Pediatrics*, **62,** 890.

Drugs and Therapeutics Bulletin (1979). Medicoal effervescent activated charcoal in the treatment of acute poisoning. *Drug. Ther. Bull.*, **17,** 7.

Easom, J.M. and Lovejoy, F.H. (1979). Efficacy and safety of gastrointestinal decontamination in the treatment of oral poisoning. *Pediatr. Clin. N. Am.*, **26,** 827.

Moore, R.A., Rumack, B.H., Conner, C.S. and Peterson, R.G. (1980). Naloxone: Underdosage after narcotic poisoning. *Am. J. Dis. Child.* **134,** 156.

Muir, I. F. K. and Barclay, T. L. (1974). *Burns and their Treatment*. Lloyd-Luke, London.

Rumack, B.H. and Matthews, H. (1975). Acetaminophen poisoning and toxicity. *Pediatrics*, **55,** 871.

Rumack, B.H. and Peterson, R.G. (1978). Acetaminophen overdose: incidence, diagnosis and management in 416 patients. *Pediatrics*, **62,** 898.

Vale, J.A. and Meredith, T.J. (ed). (1981) *Poisoning*. Update Books, London.

CHAPTER 15

Child abuse

Perhaps the single most important factor in recognizing child abuse is to be aware. In spite of the media publicity which surrounds particular cases, it remains difficult to deal personally with the clinical situation. The concept of parents inflicting damage on a child is unpleasant and it is only by recognizing and facing up to one's own feelings about this that one can become receptive and able to help these unfortunate families.

Extent of child abuse

The incidence of nonaccidental injury (NAI) is difficult to determine. The spectrum of child abuse is much wider than the physical injuries originally recognized (Figure 1) and includes neglect, emotional deprivation and sexual abuse. The definition also depends on the prevailing opinion of what behaviour is morally and socially acceptable. A survey in northeast Wiltshire analysing the number of children under four years old who had suffered severe physical abuse, revealed a rate of 1 per 1000 (Oliver *et al.*, 1974). Projection of this survey to England and Wales as a whole gives an estimate of 3000 children under four years old very severely injured each year. If other forms of abuse are also included, the number increases to at least 4 out of every 1000 children per year. It is estimated that there are 100 deaths from child abuse in the UK each year. The greatest risk of severe

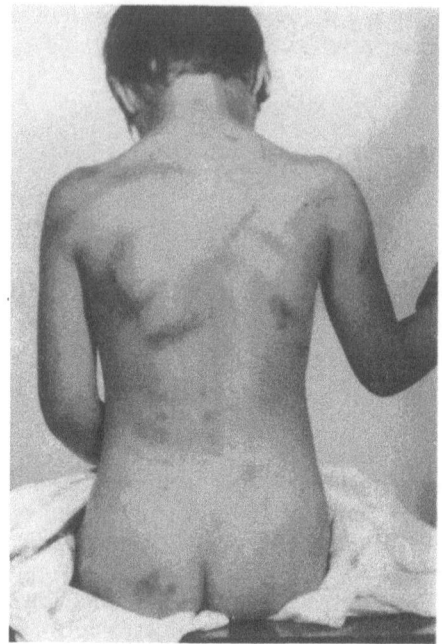

Figure 1   *Severe physical injuries are only one of the many forms of child abuse*

physical injury is to children in the first year of life with a sharp decrease as they get older.

Background

A combination of factors are usually involved in any episode of nonaccidental injury. Henry Kempe, who in 1961 forced the medical profession and the public to appreciate the magnitude of what he emotively termed the 'battered child' syndrome, has suggested that three aspects are significant in the background of most incidents: the parent's problems, the particular child and a crisis which culminates in abuse (Figure 2).

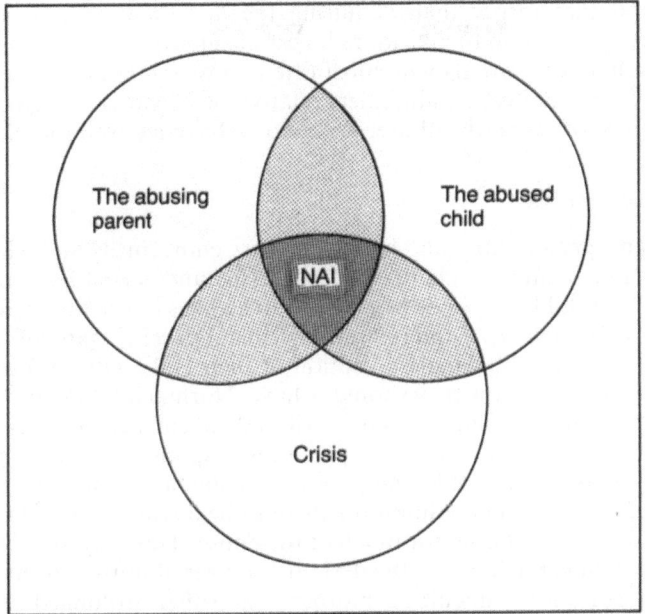

Figure 2   *Circumstances which may lead to child abuse*

The abusing parent

Abusing parents may come from all walks of life, both educated and uneducated, rich or poor. There is a fine balance between the degree of stress under which a family live and their ability to tolerate it. Poor health, poverty, poor housing, isolation from family or an unfamiliar cultural background can all act as aggravating factors. Although there is no single psychological picture in parents who abuse their children a recurring pattern is seen, in the cycle of deprivation which is passed from one generation to the next. Many of the parents are emotionally immature, having come themselves from a physically or emotionally deprived background. They often have low self-esteem, have never learned to trust or be trusted and find relationships difficult to make and maintain. Their responses are quick and intense to any kind of rejection, whether real or imaginary. They may search for love at any price, marrying and having their children young but then find that rather than acquiring the love they seek they are themselves called on to give more love and support.

Although it is parents who most often abuse their children, occasionally a cohabitee, childminder, relative or friend is involved. In about 10% of cases, the abuser is found to have a psychotic illness.

The abused child

Children's personalities and behaviour vary enormously and while a mother may manage a child who feeds easily and is healthy, a more demanding child who feeds reluctantly and wakes frequently at night may provoke a volatile and potentially violent parent. Many of these parents have an abnormal perception of their child with unrealistic expectations as to how they should behave. Normal infant behaviour such as crying or soiling is seen as wilful disobedience and physical punishment is regarded as an appropriate response. A mother may see her child as unlovable and gain no satisfaction from caring for his needs. It is not uncommon for there to be a scapegoat child in a family, who is the target for much of the abuse. This may arise if the child was unwanted, not of the desired sex, or is abnormal or handicapped. It is more difficult for mothers who suffer prolonged separation from sick or premature babies to form a normal maternal bond with them and these babies are at greater risk of nonaccidental injury.

The crisis

In most incidents of abuse there has been a trigger. This is often relatively trivial but causes sudden loss of control in the parent. The child's persistent crying or an incident of soiling may be seen as accusatory and arouse intolerable anxiety and frustration. The crisis may be an external event such as loss of a job or loss of a supporting friend. An important and frequent observation in cases of nonaccidental injury is the isolation of the parents. In a crisis they have no relatives or friends to whom they can turn for help, and because of their low self-esteem frequently do not believe others would want to help them.

250

Physical injuries

Presentation

Physical injuries are the commonest form of child abuse seen in the casualty department. The vast majority of injuries are from genuine accidents, but they must be differentiated from those which are deliberately inflicted. There may be clues in the history or the nature of the injury which should arouse suspicion of child abuse, and these will be described in some detail.

As those responsible for the care of children have become increasingly aware of child abuse, more cases are now referred directly to paediatric departments by health visitors, nurseries, play groups and school teachers as well as family practitioners. Other cases may be discovered after neighbours report their suspicions to social services or the NSPCC. Occasionally parents will openly seek help themselves either after hurting their child or because they are afraid they may do so.

History

In a busy casualty department it is all too easy to focus one's attention on deciding whether or not an injury needs treatment and the best form of therapy, and if none is required, simply to reassure the parent and send them home. It is vital with injuries in children, particularly babies and toddlers, to understand exactly how an accident happened. Furthermore, unless one questions not only how but why an accident occurred and what were the surrounding circumstances, cases of child abuse will be missed.

There may be features in the history which arouse suspicion. The most common clue is a discrepancy between the injury and the proposed explanation. Another is delay in reporting an injury which has clearly been present for some time. There may also be inconsistencies on repetition of the history or between different members of the family. Usually there is collusion between the family members but this may be suggested by observing their reactions during the interview. It is also useful to try to assess the parents' reactions to the injury and to the interview; do these seem appropriate or are the parents vague, elusive, unconcerned or perhaps excessively distressed, agitated or aggressive. Although older children can talk about the injury they will seldom relate the circumstances to a strange adult, although they may do so later in a less threatening environment.

If the child or siblings have been brought frequently to casualty because of injuries this should also be a warning signal.

Examination

Accidents are extremely common in children and scratches and bruises can be found on most young children. It can be very difficult to know which are outside the normal range but there are certain patterns of injuries which suggest they have been inflicted deliberately.

Bruises

Nearly all seriously injured children have had previous warning signs of bruises and minor injuries. Babies seldom incur bruises themselves and physical punishment is entirely inappropriate at this age. Any bruises, particularly of the face or head of a nonmobile baby, are suspect. Normal toddlers are often bruised but they usually bruise themselves on the extensor surfaces such as the forehead, knees and shins. Any child with multiple small injuries, especially of the face, mouth and head and particularly if they appear to have been inflicted at different times, should be viewed carefully. The shape and distribution of bruises or lacerations may clearly reflect that a child has been beaten and may suggest the object used. The severity of a child's injuries may not reflect the severity of the abuse to which they have been subjected but is more dependent on how sharp or hard an object they were struck with or thrown against.

Bruises from finger tips may be seen from gripping with excessive force (Figure 3). They are round or oval, often with the opposing thumb mark some distance away. They are mostly seen on the trunk, from shaking a child, on the proximal parts of the limbs when a child is forcibly held, or around the mouth when the cheeks are grabbed to force a baby to stop crying. The cheek is a site which is normally spared bruising, as a fall onto a flat surface results in bruising over the zygoma or chin. In a baby, it is a particularly unusual site of accidental injury.

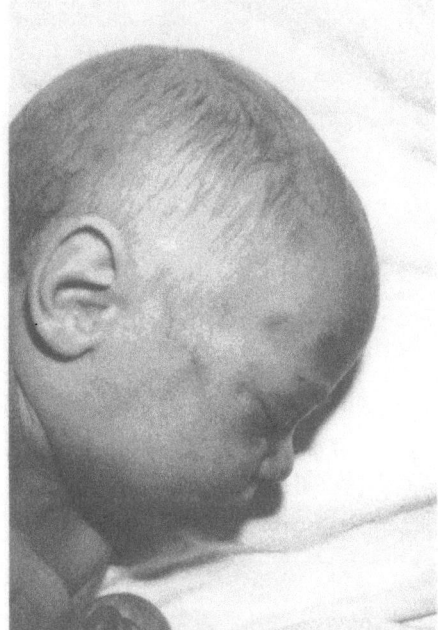

Figure 3 *Bruising from fingertips on a baby's head*

The mouth

Injuries to the mouth are common in children subjected to abuse. A torn frenulum (Figure 4) and bruising of the lips or gums should be sought in every case. They are usually caused by forcing a feeding bottle into the mouth, or from a punch.

The ear

A purple ear with petechial haemorrhages within the pinna and bruising behind the ear, is rarely seen in accidents, but usually results from a blow with the hand or fist (Figure 5).

Black eyes

Black eyes may be associated with a large bruise on the forehead or a fractured skull incurred from an accident. Otherwise, they must be

253

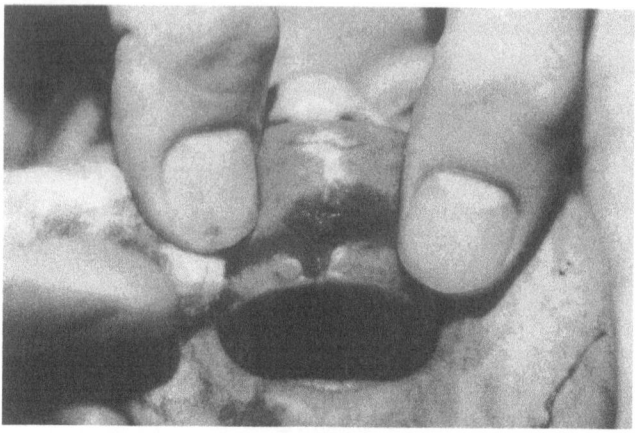

Figure 4 *The frenulum has been torn and there are tooth marks from a blow to the mouth of an eight-month-old infant*

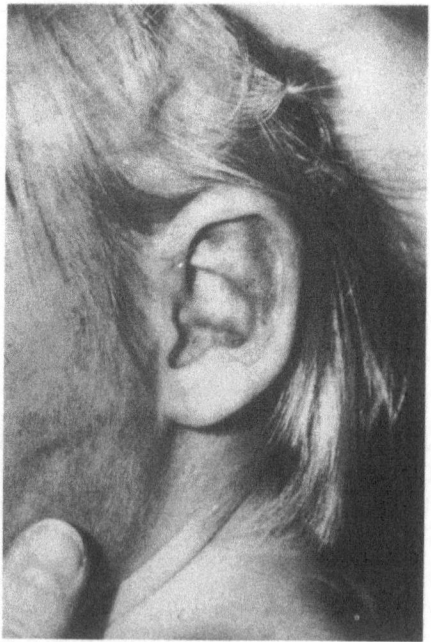

Figure 5 *Bruising within the pinna is rare in accidental injury*

caused by an object which is small enough to fit into the bony margin of the orbit, but not small enough to damage the eyeball. They are often caused by a fist or boot. Any fall onto a flat surface will bruise only the bony margins, and this makes isolated black eyes particularly suspect.

Genitalia

Lesions of the genitalia and perineal area are unusual and only rarely accidental.

Bites

Adult bites are characteristically two semicircular bruises with a gap at either end, but sometimes the bruise is a full circle (Figure 6). Siblings, especially toddlers, may use their teeth in self-defence or to

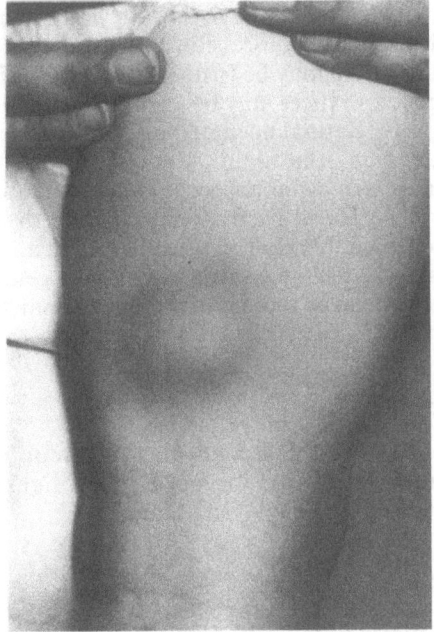

Figure 6   *A bite mark on an infant's leg*

assert themselves, but the size of their jaw is very much smaller. In cases of difficulty a dental surgeon may be able to advise.

Head injuries

Head injuries occur either from direct blows to the head or more commonly from whiplash injuries. Many mothers shake their babies in anger, thinking this is less serious than hitting their baby. This may rupture the small vessels crossing the subdural space from the brain to the dura, causing a subdural haematoma, which is responsible for most of the brain damage seen in nonaccidental injury. A similar injury, also from rapid deceleration of the head, may happen if the child's head is hit against a soft object like a bed. In neither case will there be any signs of bruising on the surface of the skull, nor any skull fracture. Intracerebral haemorrhages may accompany these injuries.

If the subdural haematoma increases in size rapidly, the infant may develop a full fontanelle, a reduced level of consciousness and convulsions. If it expands more slowly, with the development of a subdural effusion, there may be irritability, feeding difficulties, vomiting and lethargy, and there may be an abnormally rapid increase in head circumference. Retinal haemorrhages are often present and are a most important sign of head injury in child abuse. Bone fractures, especially the ribs, are often an accompanying feature in many of these children. A subdural haematoma may kill the child, or leave him mentally retarded, blind or physically disabled.

Direct blows of the head against a hard object generally cause less of a diagnostic problem as there is bruising and sometimes an underlying skull fracture.

Visceral injuries

Abdominal injuries are the second most common cause of death after brain injury. There may be no external signs of abdominal bruising from a blow to the relaxed abdomen.

Burns and scalds

It can be particularly difficult to identify burns and scalds inflicted deliberately, and the history must be carefully matched to the clinical

256

findings. Burns and scalds may be inflicted as punishment, with lesions on the buttocks and perineum particularly associated with soiling or potty training (Figure 7). Another form of punishment is with the lighted end of a cigarette, when the burns caused are small, circular and of varying depth.

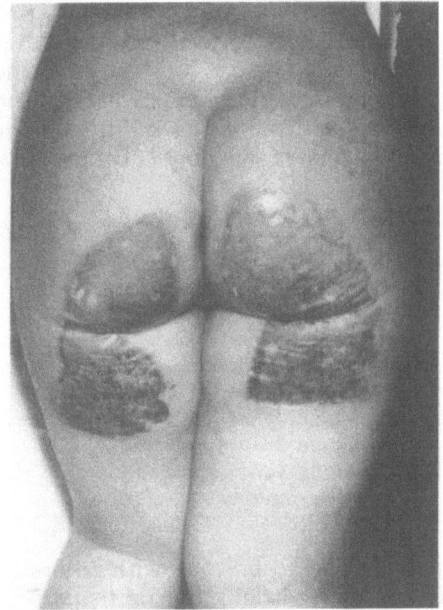

Figure 7   *Burns from sitting on a hotplate. It may have been an accident, but deliberately forcing the child to sit on the hotplate as a form of punishment was more likely*

Radiological features

In spite of the absence of clinical signs, radiological lesions are frequently seen in ill-treated infants and toddlers. Characteristically, there is radiological evidence of multiple injuries, often at different stages of healing. A midshaft fracture of a long bone in a baby not yet walking should be carefully assessed unless there is a convincing explanation. Rib fractures in a baby or toddler are rarely accidental as the ribs are compliant to all but violent blows.

Other characteristic radiographic features include epiphyseal separation from pulling a limb, and periosteal haematomas from squeezing with rotation. Evidence of healing with periosteal new bone formation may not be evident until two weeks after the injury.

Other forms of child abuse

Subtler forms of child abuse are now recognized as well as overt physical injuries. The range includes both physical and psychological neglect where children may be malnourished, forced to live in appalling conditions, suffer extreme lack of attention and stimulation, emotional deprivation and sexual abuse (Table 1).

Table 1   Forms of child abuse

Physical injury–nonaccidental
Neglect
Emotional deprivation
Sexual abuse
Other clinical disorders
    Failure to thrive
    Persistent crying and feeding problems
    Behaviour disturbance
    Poisoning
    Bizarre symptoms

The infant may present to hospital with failure to thrive, where there is failure to grow in height and particularly to gain weight. Seeking advice about vague problems of persistent crying, difficulty in feeding, or with behaviour problems, may be earlier indicators of stressed families. It may be possible to predict potential child abuse even in the maternity department when abnormal family dynamics or bonding failure are noted (Lynch and Roberts, 1977).

Other bizarre forms of child abuse are also recognized, such as deliberate poisoning by giving repeated doses of drugs such as aspirin, salt or diuretics. This may even be surreptitiously continued after the child is admitted to hospital. Parents may simulate diseases, such as diabetes by putting sugar in the child's urine, or invent symptoms so that the child has repeated investigations. Whenever children present with peculiar unexplainable symptoms child abuse should be considered.

Admission to hospital

If nonaccidental injury is suspected either in the community or in hospital, a paediatrician should be contacted and in most cases the child admitted to hospital. If sympathetically handled, most parents are willing to accept medical advice that their child needs to be admitted for observation and investigations. This will ensure that the child is in a safe environment with experienced staff who are available at all times. In addition, any injuries or medical conditions can be identified and treated, and alternative diagnoses excluded (Figure 8). Occasionally parents cannot be persuaded to accept the child's admission to hospital. If the child's safety is considered to be at risk, a Place of Safety Order will be required (see Appendix).

Initial assessment in the hospital should be made preferably by a

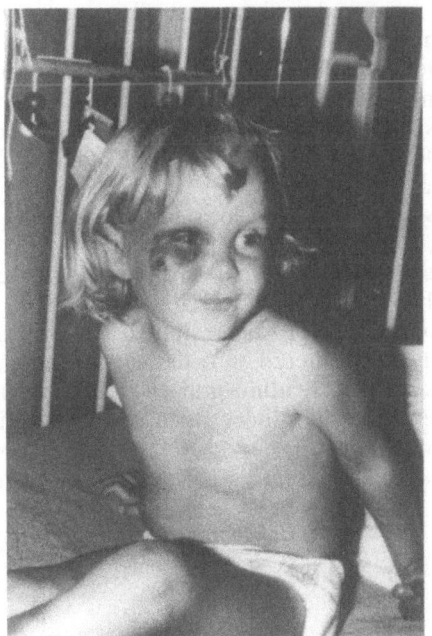

Figure 8 *Children with suspected nonaccidental injury need a thorough medical examination. Abuse was suspected in this girl as this large bruise followed what was said to be a minor bump. She had multiple bruises and a few petechiae, and had idiopathic thrombocytopenic purpura*

senior member of the paediatric staff with experience in cases of child abuse. A thorough history should be taken in a sensitive and concerned way, without being accusatory or condemning. It is generally unhelpful and unproductive to try to seek a confession. This assessment requires time to assemble a picture not only of the circumstances surrounding any injury, but also of the social background and family dynamics. This includes discovering from parents how they see themselves, each other and their child, how they deal with difficult behaviour and how they punish their children.

When the child is examined, preferably with the parents present, the child's mood and interactions with his parents can be observed.

Many of the physical signs of abuse have already been described, and examination inside the mouth and of the fundi must not be omitted. In addition to noting the child's state of hygiene, the height and weight is measured and an overall assessment of the child's development made.

Detailed notes must be taken, preferably using the parents' own words. Diagrams and photographs must be made of any injuries.

If NAI is suspected, a skeletal survey should be performed. Single radiographs of the whole body are best avoided as they do not provide optimal views of individual bones, and individual radiographs of the skull, chest, and long bones including the hands and feet are required. As very recent injuries may not be evident, radiographs may need to be repeated two weeks later or a bone scan performed. When radiographic abnormalities are present, underlying bone disorders need to be excluded. All are rare, but the one most commonly encountered is osteogenesis imperfecta. In most cases the bones are clearly abnormal on radiographs, but it may be impossible to exclude the milder form of this condition on radiographs alone. In this disorder, fractures of the long bones involve the diaphyses and not the metaphyses. Rarely, infantile cortical hyper-

Table 2   Coagulation studies

Full blood count
Platelet count
Bleeding time
Prothrombin time
Partial thromboplastin time
Thrombin time
Factor VIII assay in selected cases

ostosis (Caffey's disease), osteomyelitis, scurvy, congenital syphilis and rickets need to be considered. When there are unexplained bruises, clotting studies will be required (Table 2).

In addition to the medical assessment, social workers and professionals from other disciplines will need to evaluate the parents and the family situation, and initiate support and guidance as appropriate. The police may also be involved.

Case conference

A case conference should be convened promptly with all those who can contribute background information, provide specialist expertise or offer assistance. This may include, in addition to the paediatric staff, the hospital and local authority social workers, NSPCC personnel, general practitioner, health visitors, teachers, psychiatrist, juvenile bureau, police and any other agencies involved with the family concerned. While the team is assembled and its members are accumulating information for the case conference, the child should be kept in hospital.

There are many difficulties in managing large case conferences, including relying on participants being well-informed and providing only relevant information. In spite of the problems they are of great value in dealing with these complex situations. Several decisions need to be taken. The first is to decide if this really is a case of nonaccidental injury. If so, plans need to be made regarding the child's safety—whether he can return home under supervision or if it is necessary to remove the child from his parents and place him in the care of others, either on a voluntary basis, or if necessary, by legal proceedings. A key-worker will need to be designated, usually a social worker from the NSPCC or local authority. Each health authority keeps an 'at risk' register, and whether the child and any siblings should be placed on it must also be decided. A review procedure should be instituted and long-term plans made regarding the nature and extent of social work involvement, and if medical surveillance is required.

The broad objectives of management are for babies and children to be protected from any further physical injury and for them to live in an environment where they can grow and develop optimally. The aim is for the family to be rehabilitated whenever this is a practical possibility. While it is simple to assert these general objectives, achieving them can be extremely difficult, and makes huge demands on personnel and money. Sometimes it is impossible to meet these expectations, particularly as some of the most serious problems arise in families who are not accessible to help. In the long term, the management of child abuse lies not in crisis intervention, important as this is, but rather in moulding the attitudes of society to the welfare of children.

References

Lynch, M.A. and Roberts J. (1977). *Br. Med. J.*, **1**, 624.

Oliver, J.E., Cox, J., Taylor, A. and Baldwin, J.A. (1974). *Severely ill-treated young children in northeast Wiltshire*, Oxford Unit of Clinical Epidemiology, University Research Report No. 4.

Further reading

Kempe, R.S. and Kempe, C.H. (1978). *Child Abuse*, Fontana/Open Books, London.

Kempe, C.H. and Helfer, R.E. (1972) (Eds). *Helping the Battered Child and his Family*, J.B. Lippincott, Philadelphia.

Lee, C.M. (Ed) (1978). *Child Abuse, a Reader and Sourcebook*, Open University Press, Milton Keynes.

Smith, S.M. (1978) (Ed). *The Maltreatment of Children*, MTP Press Ltd., Lancaster.

Note

In England, any person (usually a social worker or NSPCC inspector) may apply for a Place of Safety Order (an Order under Section 28 of the Children and Young Persons Act 1969). The applicant must convince a magistrate that a child's proper development is being avoidably prevented or neglected or his health is being avoidably impaired or neglected and he is being ill-treated. Once the Order has been made the child may be detained in a 'place of safety', for example, a hospital, for a maximum of 28 days.

CHAPTER 16

Sudden infant death syndrome

Incidence, definition and aetiology

About 1500 infants die suddenly and unexpectedly in the UK each year, making this the commonest cause of death in infants aged between four weeks and one year. This means that one in 500 apparently healthy babies will die from SIDS. The peak incidence is at two to four months, but there is a wide range extending from a few days old to two years (Figure 1). Typically, the infant is put to bed at night and found dead in the morning. It happens quietly and not uncommonly while the parents are asleep in the same bedroom. The incidence is highest in autumn and winter when respiratory illness is prevalent in the community; it is higher in boys, in low-birth-weight infants, in babies who are bottle fed, when the mother is young and when the socioeconomic circumstances are poor. However, contrary to popular belief, victims come from all social classes and include those who have been wholly breast fed.

The term 'cot death' is often used in the UK, while the expression 'sudden infant death syndrome' is used in North America and in the paediatric literature. It has been defined as the sudden death of any infant which is unexpected from the history and where a thorough autopsy fails to demonstrate an adequate cause of death. (Beckwith, 1970) This definition is not precise, as it leaves unanswered what constitutes a thorough post-mortem and what is considered to be an adequate cause of death.

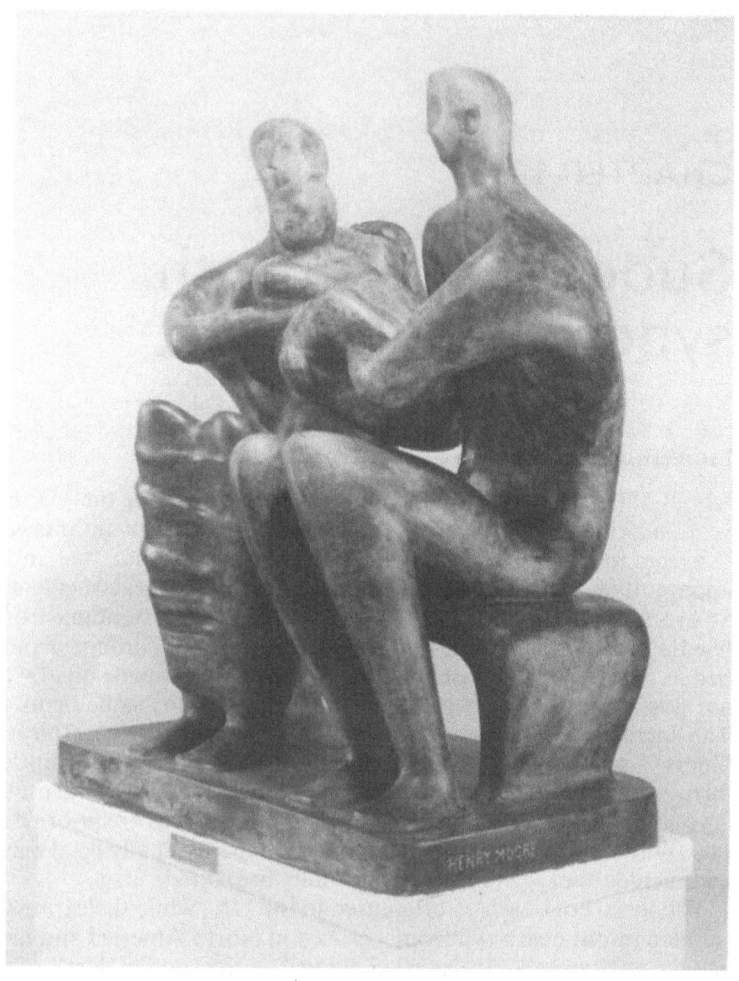

'Family Group' by Sir Henry Moore. A baby is the centre of the family's attention, making a cot death particularly tragic and hard to bear. © *Copyright Tate Gallery, London*

264

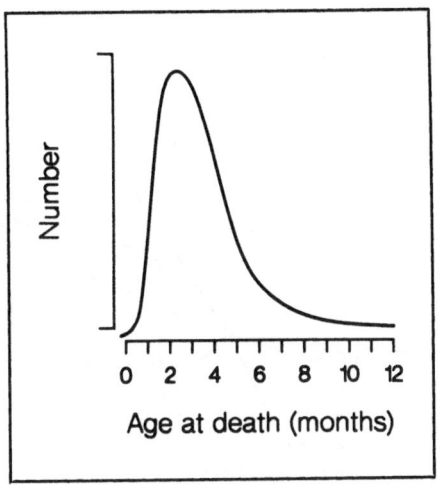

Figure 1 *Age distribution of sudden unexpected deaths*

In fact, many infants who die suddenly and unexpectedly from the history have not died from sudden infant death syndrome according to this definition. A study at autopsy of all children who died suddenly and unexpectedly in the Sheffield area showed that one-third had evidence of gross disease, such as pneumonia, meningitis or hypernatraemic dehydration following gastroenteritis. A second large group had evidence of minor disease such as tracheobronchitis which was thought to be insufficient in itself to have been the cause of death. The third and smallest group showed no significant abnormalities, only the nonspecific findings of widespread petechiae over the lungs and some alveolar oedema and congestion (Figure 2). A few of these infants will have died of non-accidental injury. Most of these have evidence of gross disease, in particular subdural haematomas, but in some no significant abnormality can be detected at autopsy.

Numerous theories have been proposed to explain the causes of SIDS. (Table 1). Rather than a single cause there appear to be several contributing factors.

Clinical investigation has revealed that while it is often said that these infants have been perfectly well, in fact many experience a

265

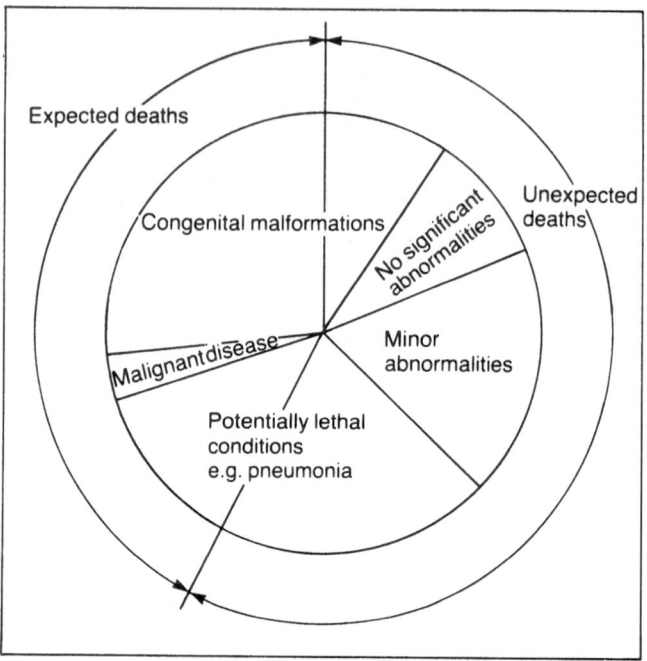

Figure 2 *Autopsy findings of infants aged between one week and one year in Sheffield in 1972 and 1973 (adapted from Emery, 1976)*

Table 1 **Some theories which have been proposed to explain the causes of the sudden infant death syndrome**

Respiratory	Abnormal ventilatory control
	apnoea
	chronic hypoxia
	Upper airways obstruction
Cardiac	Dysrhythmia or conduction disturbances
Infection	Viral illnesses
Immunological	Hypersensitivity to specific proteins
Nutritional deficiency	
Subclinical abnormality	Metabolic
	Brain damage
Hyperthermia	
Sociological factors	

266

variety of symptoms before their deaths. Most are nonspecific, such as irritability, drowsiness or mild coryzal symptoms. A retrospective survey showed that 59% of infants had experienced symptoms during the last few days of their life (Stanton *et al.*, 1978).

Detailed postmortem examination has also revealed that in many cases there is evidence that the infant has not been thriving for some time. This is suggested by gross disturbances in the bones and fatty changes in the liver (Sinclair-Smith *et al.*, 1976). Evidence from one centre suggests that in some cases there is hypertrophy of the musculature of the pulmonary arteries suggesting that they have suffered from chronic hypoxia (Naeye, 1980). It has been postulated that chronic underventilation occurs during sleep.

Most attention is currently focussed on apnoea. Evidence is accumulating that abnormalities of ventilatory control may be important and that prolonged apnoea is likely to be the final event in some cases of sudden infant death syndrome (*British Medical Journal*, 1980). As mentioned above, infants who die unexpectedly have often had preceding coryzal symptoms and many have mucosal changes indicating the presence of viral upper respiratory tract infection. Some infants with only mild upper respiratory infections have been shown to develop periodic respiration which is accompanied by prolonged periods of apnoea.

There is also evidence to suggest that there is a certain group of infants who have a particularly poor ventilatory drive, who may be at increased risk of cot deaths. Continuous monitoring of children who have had near-misses of sudden death—who have been found apnoeic and been resuscitated—has shown that some of them experience prolonged periods of apnoea even without evidence of intercurrent infection (Southall *et al.*, 1980). It has been suggested that infants die of sudden infant death syndrome when certain predisposing factors coincide. These may include abnormal ventilatory control, cardiac dysrhythmias, certain sleep patterns and viral infections. The ultimate aim of this research is to be able to identify infants at risk and make prevention possible.

Accident and emergency department

Cardiorespiratory resuscitation of an infant found apparently dead in his cot will usually be started by the ambulance crew and then continued by the medical staff after arrival at the hospital. While resuscitation is in progress, it is important to obtain an accurate history from the parent or whoever has rushed the infant to the accident and emergency department. It is also useful to find out the name of the general practitioner and if there has been close involvement by a health visitor or any other community health workers. If only one parent is present, the other parent, a relative, or friend should be contacted.

If resuscitation is unsuccessful the doctor in charge will have to decide before interviewing the parents whether sudden infant death syndrome was the most likely cause of death. This requires evaluating the history and checking that there are no signs of injury or disease. Few investigations are worthwhile, but a blood culture from an intracardiac blood sample may very occasionally yield useful information.

The parents

Telling the parents that their small baby has died can only be a painful and difficult task for any doctor. Most parents are initially overwhelmed with shock and bewilderment by their sudden loss and many find it impossible to believe that their baby has really died. After explaining that their child has most probably died from the sudden infant death syndrome, the parents need to know that a postmortem will have to be performed to establish the cause of death with greater certainty. Many parents are upset by this and will be even more distressed when they are told that the coroner has to be informed. They will be interviewed by the police who will ask questions about the circumstances leading to their infant's death and an inquest may be held. The coroner is associated in most people's minds with criminal proceedings, and it must be emphasized that it does not in any way mean that they are suspected of a criminal act or that they were the cause of their infant's death.

Many parents rapidly recall the past events and search for possible causes for their child's death. Many are afraid that they were in some way responsible for their infant's death or might have prevented it. The nature of SIDS needs to be explained and any mistaken preconceived notions corrected. It should be emphasized that they were in no way responsible for the death and that it is unrelated to sleeping position, suffocation or feeding habits. Many parents experience strong feelings of guilt and self-recrimination and they need to be

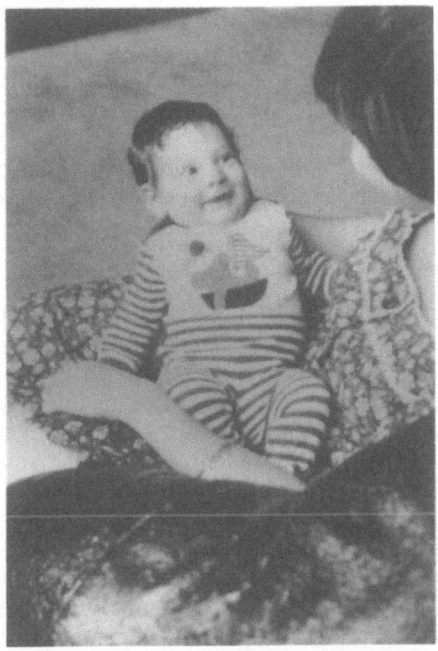

The strong bonding between a mother and her child makes most mothers feel guilty for their baby's death

reassured that these are natural but unfounded. It the death occurred when a relative or baby-sitter was looking after the infant, such feelings of guilt by both parties involved can be particularly difficult to contain.

Many parents want to hold their baby and say 'good-bye' and they should be encouraged and offered the opportunity to do this. Death is no longer a part of everyday life and most people have never seen a dead person. Parents who do not have a real image of their dead baby may experience added unnecessary distress as a result of their fantasies. Holding their dead baby in their arms may help them acknowledge the reality of the death, and the memory can be of value to them during the subsequent period of intense mourning. Some parents wish to see a minister of religion.

A copy of the leaflet 'Information for the parent of a child who

269

has died suddenly and unexpectedly in infancy' can be given to the parents. (This is available from The Foundation for the Study of Infant Deaths, 5th Floor, 5 Grosvenor Place, London SW1X 7HD, tel. 01-235 1721.) Through the Foundation parents can be put into contact with other parents who live in the same area and who have been through a similar experience, and they can also obtain further information about the sudden infant death syndrome.

Further care

The general practitioner needs to be informed so that he can provide guidance and support for the family during this difficult period. Parents experience intense grief reactions which may include hallucinations of seeing their baby or hearing his cries. Warning parents of the possible reactions and reassuring them that they are normal and will eventually fade may be helpful to them. Advice may also be sought by parents regarding other siblings. Explaining the baby's death honestly to the other children is important and the intensity of their grief and fantasies—which will depend on their age—may surprise their parents. Initiated by their normal jealousy of a new baby, older children may feel they were in some way responsible for the death. Honest discussion and acknowledgement of feelings of guilt and sadness between the members of the family will help maintain family unity.

A social worker, especially if already involved with the family, and the health visitor should be contacted so that they can also give support if required.

The role of the paediatrician

It is valuable if the parents can be seen by the consultant paediatrician immediately, and again two to three weeks later. This will enable the results of the postmortem to be discussed and offer another opportunity for the parents to ask questions and express their feelings. By then the parents will have been given the death certificate by the coroner's officer stating the cause of death. Many coroners continue to be unwilling to mention sudden infant death syndrome on the death certificate even when no adequate cause of death can be found and they will give a cause such as 'viral pneumonitis' instead. This is likely to cause further confusion for the family, particularly after all

the explanations of the inconclusive state of knowledge of the aetiology of SIDS.

It is often on this occasion that the parents will enquire about the
risks for siblings and any further children. Older children are not at
risk, but the risk for a twin is considerable (4%) and warrants immediate and careful evaluation. For subsequent children the risk is
increased ten-fold, but it is highly unlikely for there to be a second
occurrence within the same family. Parents can thus be reassured
that the chance of a recurrence is small, at 2 in 100 (Peterson,
1980).

There has been considerable controversy over the use of apnoea
monitors at home for subsequent children. Looking after a child at
home who is monitored 24 hours a day for several months raises
many technical problems and extra emotional strain for the parents
and everyone else looking after the baby. The widespread use of
home monitoring cannot be advocated at present, considering the
current state of knowledge and the monitors at present on the market.
Facilities are available for a single 24 hour electrocardiographic and
respiratory tracing to be made, and this can be done while the infant
is at home. The technique may possibly enable a markedly abnormal
pattern of breathing or a cardiac dysrhythmia to be detected and
treated.

Contact with the family should be maintained over a long period
by the paediatrician and general practitioner. After the initial shock,
there is usually a prolonged period of grief and mourning in the
family. A further pregnancy is often accompanied by fears of a
recurrence, coupled with considerable anxiety and doubt on the
parents' part as to their ability to cope with the new baby. Even
minor illnesses suffered by subsequent babies may cause panic. Tension often runs high as the child approaches the age when the previous infant died. Once beyond this age a major milestone has been
passed.

Although many doctors find it difficult and uncomfortable to deal
with the feelings of a bereaved family, a cot death should not result
in a single encounter between the paediatrician or general practitioner and the infant's parents, but should initiate a long term relationship with the family.

References

Beckwith, J.B. (1970), in *SIDS: Proceedings of the second International Conference on Causes of Sudden Deaths in Infants*, Bergman, A.B., Beckwith, J.B., Ray, C. (Ed.) University of Washington Press, Seattle. p. 83.

British Medical Journal (1980), Sudden infant death syndrome and ventilatory control, **281**, 337.

Naeye, R.L. (1980), *Scientific American*, **242**, 4, 52.

Peterson, D.R. (1980), *J. Pediatr.*, **97**, 265.

Sinclair-Smith, C., Dinsdale, F. and Emery, J.L. (1976), *Arch. Dis. Child.*, **51**, 424.

Southall, D.P., Richards, J., Brown, D.J., Johnston, P.G.B., de Swiet, H. and Shinebourne, E.A. (1980), *Arch. Dis. Child*, **55**, 7.

Stanton, A.N., Downham, M.A.P.S., Oakley, J.R., Emery, J.L. and Knowelden, J. (1978), *Br. Med. J.*, **2**, 1249.

Further reading

Emery, J.L. (1976), Unexpected death in infancy, in *Recent Advances in Paediatrics*, Hull, D. (ed.), Churchill Livingstone, Edinburgh.

Emery, J.L. (1979), Cot death, *J. Matern. Child Health*, **4**, 374

Limerick, Lady S. (1979), Counselling parents who have experienced a cot death in the family. *J. Matern. Child Health*, **4**, 438.

Meadow, R. (1982), Munchausen syndrome by proxy. *Arch. Dis. Child.*, **57**, 92.

Moore, A. (1981), The sudden infant death syndrome, *Br. J. Hosp. Med.*, **26**, 5, 37.

CHAPTER 17

Practical procedures

Practical procedures are most easily learnt by observation and then practice. There are many ways in which any procedure may be performed and the methods described here are those of personal preference. In paediatrics considerable time is spent on practical procedures and each unsuccessful attempt is traumatic not only for the child but also for the parents, doctors and assistants.

Most procedures are more difficult in babies and infants than in adults because of their smaller size, and their inability to co-operate. It is essential to be well organized before starting, with all the apparatus assembled, strips of tape cut and specimen containers to hand. An experienced assistant is of prime importance in the success of any procedure. The child should be held as comfortably as possible but restrained sufficiently to avoid jeopardizing the procedure.

It is generally best to have a flexible attitude as to whether the child's parents should be present during the procedure and to discuss the matter freely with them. Some children are very anxious for their parents' support, and whilst some parents are particularly keen to stay others are uncomfortable with the situation and prefer to wait outside. The nature of the procedure and one's own confidence in coping with the parents' presence should also be considered. It is not advisable to ask parents to restrain their children or act as an assistant as their role should be to give support and encouragement to their child.

It is easy to forget that even young children need to know what is going to happen to them. It is important to be honest and not to say something will not hurt if it does. Talking to the children during the procedure is reassuring and often they will appreciate knowing what they should do to help – for example that it is important to try and keep still but that it doesn't matter if they cry. It is worth enquiring what in particular worries them, as children's fears are frequently different from adults, and then the reassurance can be appropriate. A 5 ml syringe of blood may seem immense to a 5-year-old with no concept of his total blood volume and telling him he has plenty of blood left may help him considerably.

For procedures which are particularly painful or frightening, or if several procedures need to be performed at the same time it is kinder to sedate the child (Table 1) or to give a general anaesthetic. After

Table 1   Some sedatives used for practical procedures in young children

Age	Drug
< 1 year	Chloral hydrate p.o. 30–50 mg/kg to max. of 1 g or Trimeprazine (Vallergan) p.o. 2–4 mg/kg
1–5 years	Trimeprazine (Vallergan) p.o. 4 mg/kg to max. of 120 mg ± Droperidol p.o. 1.25–2.5 mg or Omnopon 0.4 mg/kg + Hyoscine (Scopalamine) 8 µg/kg ⎫ i.m. to maximum of 20 mg Omnopon or Diazepam (Valium) 0.2 mg/kg slow i.v. (monitor for respiratory depression)

sedation only the gentlest restraint should be necessary. A standard regimen to ensure adequate sedation cannot be given as the depth of sedation required will depend on the procedure performed and there is a very wide variation in response between different children to the same dose of sedative. It is safest to fast children for four hours before a major procedure, especially if a general anaesthetic may be required.

If one is unsuccessful after a couple of attempts, it is best to ask a colleague for assistance.

Blood samples

Blood may be taken by capillary puncture, venepuncture or by arterial puncture. The blood volume of a neonate is only 80 ml/kg and of an infant 60–70 ml/kg and so the minimum volume of blood required should be taken.

Capillary puncture

Capillary samples can be obtained from the heel or finger. The heel is a useful site in the neonate (Figure 1). One should avoid the area

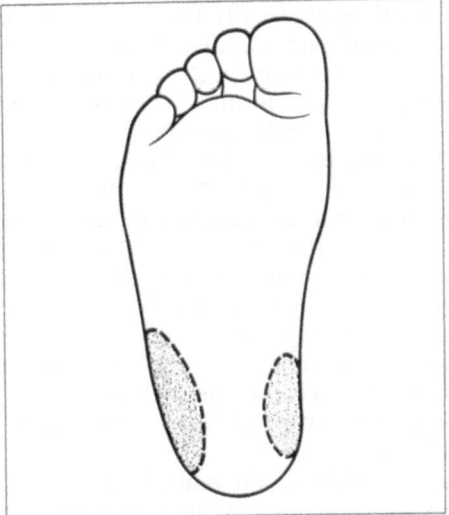

Figure 1   *Suitable sites for heel pricks*

over the Achilles tendon as the calcaneus may be pierced with the risk of osteomyelitis. It is also best to avoid sites which have already been punctured. It can be helpful to have the heel below the level of the rest of the body, and if necessary it can be warmed by holding cotton wool soaked in warm water around it for a few minutes. The foot is held dorsiflexed with the thumb and fingers around the calf and foot, and the heel protruding through the circle made by them. After cleaning the foot with an isopropyl alcohol swab, a disposable, shielded lancet is inserted about 2 mm, and the incision extended very slightly to one side. Alternatively, an Autolet, a spring-loaded device with disposable lancets can be used. To ensure that the blood will form discrete droplets, the area around the puncture can be wiped with a thin layer of sterile soft paraffin, but this is best avoided. Specially designed micropipettes or capillary tubes, lined with anticoagulant if required, facilitate the collection of capillary samples. Alternatively, the drops can be collected into small containers, tapping them periodically so that the blood mixes with the anticoagulant. The lower leg can be gently and intermittently occluded with the fingers around the calf. Avoid squeezing the foot excessively or tissue fluid will be squeezed out. Results are less reliable than from venepuncture, but there is usually reasonable correlation between capillary and venous samples. Capillary haematocrits are higher than venous, and plasma potassium results tend to be artificially raised from haemolysis. Any significantly abnormal results should be checked with a venous sample. Capillary samples are particularly useful for serial measurements of blood glucose and bilirubin levels, and also for Guthrie tests. Up to 2 ml of blood may be obtained from capillary samples but venepuncture is required if larger samples are needed or for coagulation studies or blood cultures. In neonates, if the feet are warm and peripheral perfusion is good, capillary blood gases can be estimated. A good free flow of blood needs to be obtained, without squeezing. The arterial oxygen tension may be underestimated by this technique but the other parameters are more reliable and it is valuable as an adjunct to continuous monitoring of the Pao_2 with a skin electrode although periodically arterial blood gases must also be measured.

In infants and older children the ventrolateral aspects of the fingers can also be used for capillary sampling. This site is convenient for blood glucose monitoring using an Autolet, and many older diabetic children will do this themselves. Although phlebotomists can obtain good samples from finger pricks, this method is seldom used by doctors.

Venepuncture

The antecubital fossa is the best site at all ages. The veins are of sufficient calibre for blood to be withdrawn without difficulty, and are not used for intravenous infusions. The child needs to be held comfortably by an assistant, who can use one hand to occlude the venous return of the child's upper arm and the other to hold the child's arm steady and supinated (Figure 2). It can be helpful to wrap

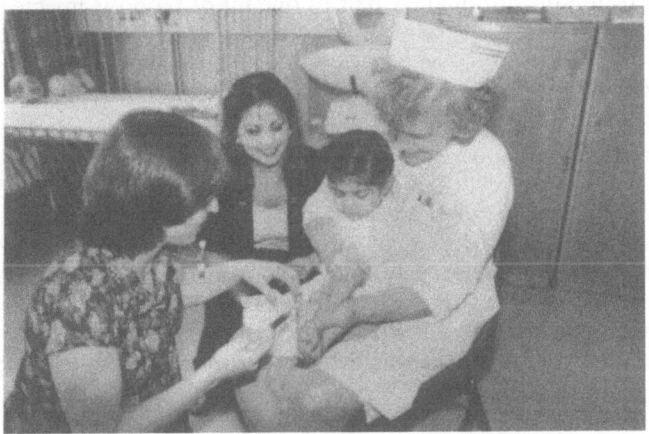

Figure 2 *Venepuncture in a young child. An experienced assistant is vital for success. The child's mother is holding his hand*

babies in a sheet or towel. In chubby or dark-skinned babies it is often possible to palpate the veins although they may not be visible. A 23G butterfly needle is suitable for babies and toddlers. The skin is cleaned with an alcohol swab, and whilst advancing the needle the skin distal to it is gently stretched to anchor the vein. If the cap at the end of the butterfly is removed, blood will flow into the tubing immediately the vein is entered. If necessary, a piece of surgical tape can be applied over the needle to keep it in position, and after attaching the syringe blood can be withdrawn by gently applying steady suction. The vessels of the back of the hands and the feet can be used, but is more difficult to withdraw blood from them. This problem can be overcome by using a standard 21G or 23G needle and letting the blood drip into the containers.

The sagittal sinus and jugular veins are not recommended as puncture sites, as the techniques are frightening for the child and the vessels are close to vital structures. The femoral vein is also best avoided apart from an emergency, as the hip joint may be entered with the risk of septic arthritis or avascular necrosis of the femoral head.

If the blood is to be cultured, the skin needs to be first cleaned with povidone–iodine, which must be allowed to dry, and a strict no-touch technique adopted. A half to one ml of blood is injected into each culture bottle.

Arterial sampling

Arterial blood samples are required for blood gas analysis, which are essential in the management of severely ill children. When the arterial oxygen tension is recorded continuously in neonates the Pao_2 drops markedly whenever a baby is disturbed, even for minor nursing procedures. If the baby cries whilst an arterial sample is obtained, the Pao_2 falls precipitiously, and inappropriate decisions may be taken in the light of these results (Figure 3). The $Paco_2$ will also be affected, but usually to a lesser degree. For this reason it is important for infants to be disturbed as little as possible whilst the sample is taken. If repeated samples are needed an arterial line can be inserted,

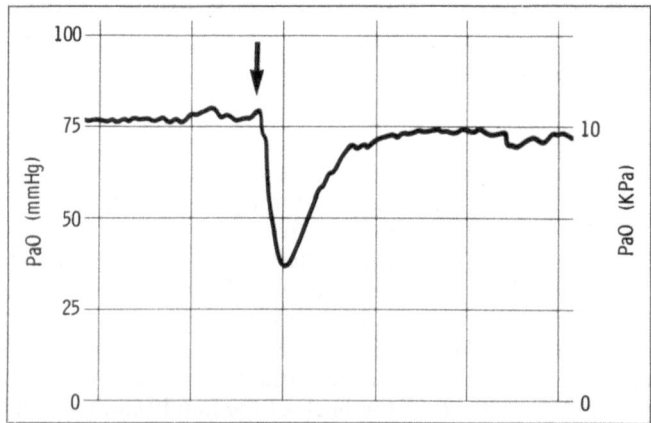

Figure 3 *Continuous recording of the Pao_2 showing the marked drop in Pao_2 during a radial artery puncture. The arrow indicates insertion of the needle*

from which repeated samples can be drawn without disturbing the child. Their main disadvantages are that insertion may be difficult, that any child with an arterial line needs to be under constant skilled nursing supervision, and that there are potentially serious complications.

Arterial puncture

The radial artery is the most common site used in children and in the neonate the right radial artery is preferred as it is preductal. Before a needle is inserted into the radial artery, the adequacy of the collateral supply must be tested by occluding both the radial and ulnar arteries. Whilst the hand is blanched, pressure on the ulnar artery is released, and flushing over the whole hand indicates that the collateral circulation is satisfactory. A short 25G needle with a 2 ml syringe attached can be used (Shaw, 1968). The syringe and needle are flushed with heparin (1000 units/ml), leaving heparin to fill the syringe dead space. In the neonate, local anaesthetic is not always used as it makes the tissues swell, making it more difficult to localize the artery and infiltration of the skin with local anaesthetic seems to cause as much discomfort as performing the arterial puncture. In infants and young children 1% plain lignocaine without adrenaline

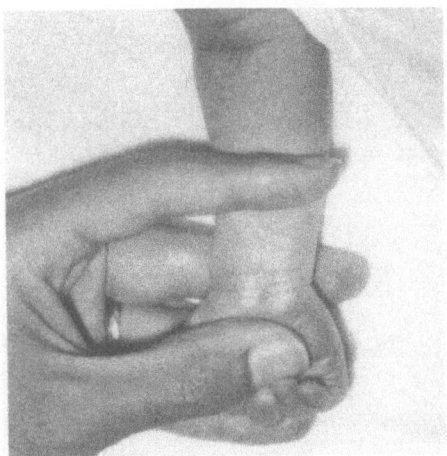

Figure 4 *Holding the arm in preparation for a radial artery puncture in a neonate*

279

should be infiltrated, and two to three minutes allowed for the anaesthetic to act and the child to settle. It is important to hold the child's hand correctly, so that the needle is not dislodged if the child moves. In the neonate and infant, this can be achieved by holding the arm in the anatomical position, with one's thumb in the palm of the baby's hand, and using the index and middle fingers to hold the arm steady (Figure 4). The wrist should not be hyperextended. The position of the artery can be determined by palpation and, in the neonate, with the bright light source of a transilluminator. The light source should not be left in contact with the skin as it may cause a burn. In the neonate, at the proximal skin crease of the wrist, the artery usually lies in the middle of the lateral third of the forearm. After cleaning the skin the needle is inserted bevel upwards along the line of the artery, at 30° to 45° to the horizontal, until one meets resistance. This means it will have gone through both walls of the artery. Very gentle suction is then applied to the plunger of the syringe and the needle is slowly withdrawn. Additional stability can be provided by resting the needle on one's other thumb (Figure 5). Blood will flow into the syringe when the tip of the needle lies in the lumen of the artery. If the initial attempt is unsuccessful, one can try again slightly to either side, without withdrawing the needle from the skin. Alternatively, a short 25G Butterfly needle can be used. It is

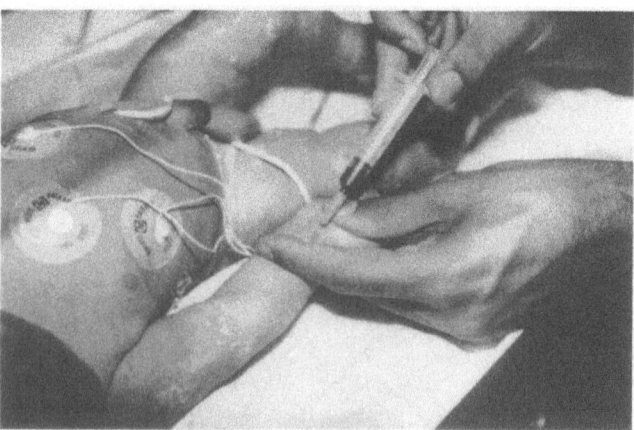

Figure 5 *Radial artery puncture with a heparinized syringe and short 25G needle*

preferable to take 0.25 ml of blood to avoid the heparin affecting the acid–base balance. A steady flow of blood is needed, without bubbles of air. Once the sample has been obtained, any air should be expelled, a cap placed on the end of the syringe and the sample analysed immediately, otherwise the sample should be kept on ice. The puncture site needs to be compressed for 3 to 5 minutes and then checked to make sure that bleeding has stopped.

Arterial catheters

The radial artery is the site most often used other than the umbilical artery in neonates. Another convenient site is the dorsalis pedis artery. The temporal artery is sometimes used in neonates but carries

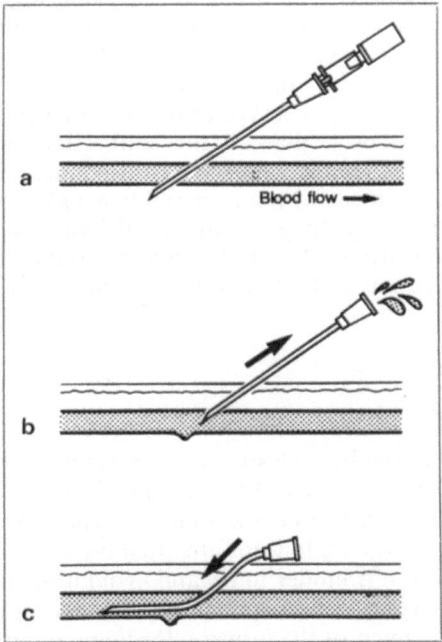

Figure 6   *Insertion of a radial artery catheter.* **a.** *The artery is transfixed with a 22G or 24G cannula.* **b.** *After removing the needle, the cannula is withdrawn until blood flows back along the cannula.* **c.** *The cannula is advanced along the lumen of the artery*

a risk of necrosis of the scalp and cerebral emboli by retrograde flow on flushing. The posterior tibial, brachial or femoral arteries are other possible sites. Before a radial artery catheter is inserted the collateral blood supply to the hand must be checked. The hand needs to be well splinted, with a role of gauze under the wrist. After cleaning the skin, local anaesthetic is infiltrated. A skin incision is made with a lancet. One technique is to use a 22G or 24G plastic cannula which is inserted to transfix the artery as described for arterial sampling (Figure 6a). The needle is removed, and the cannula slowly withdrawn. When blood flows back into the cannula (Figure 6b) the cannula is held almost horizontal and advanced with gentle rotation along the lumen of the artery (Figure 6c). Excessive blood loss can be prevented by pressing on the artery proximal to the cannula. It is also possible to cannulate an artery in the same way as a vein by advancing the cannula until it just enters the artery and then, whilst holding the needle steady, gently advancing the cannula with rotation. The cannula can be attached to a short length of extension tubing and via a 3-way tap to a syringe pump with heparinized saline. It is important to check that all the connections are firm, well strapped and can be readily observed as disconnection and exsanguination is a real danger with an arterial line. Other complications include embolism and damage to the distal blood supply, and the fingers must be clearly visible. Indwelling arterial catheters should only be used if the nurses looking after the child are experienced in their care.

Intravenous infusions

In young children, the best sites for an intravenous infusion are the veins on the back of the hands. Other sites are the feet, and sometimes the veins on the forearm and the long saphenous vein of the leg (Figure 7). In neonates, scalp veins are often used. They may also be used in infants, but it is kinder to try and avoid using the scalp, as it is usually necessary to shave a patch of hair, leaving the child and parents with the stigma of the infusion for many months. The veins in the antecubital fossa are usually avoided because of the discomfort involved in splinting the elbow, and the cannulae become kinked if the arm is flexed. Check which thumb the child sucks and if he is right- or left-handed before choosing which arm to immobilize.

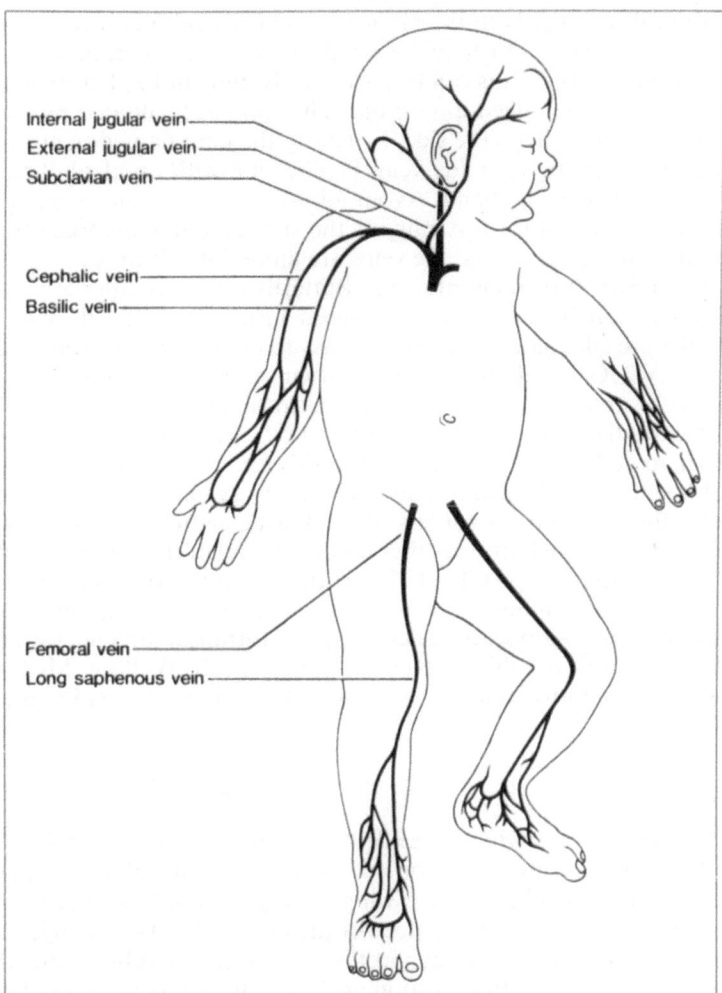

Internal jugular vein
External jugular vein
Subclavian vein

Cephalic vein
Basilic vein

Femoral vein
Long saphenous vein

Figure 7   *Veins for intravenous infusion or sampling in infants*

Peripheral infusions

All intravenous infusions in children should be given via a paediatric burette and an infusion pump to ensure that an excessive volume of fluid is not given inadvertently. These should be prepared and nearby.

283

A suitable site needs to be selected so that the calibre of the vein is sufficiently large and where the needle or cannula will be able to rest comfortably. The veins can be particularly difficult to identify in the chubby six- to eighteen-month-old. This may be facilitated by using indirect lighting from the side, by letting the limb hang downwards, by gently tapping over the vein, by cleaning with an alcohol swab and by warming the hand. Avoid allowing the assistant to occlude the venous return for too long, or the skin becomes engorged from capillary hyperaemia and the veins are more difficult to see.

For most intravenous infusions, Butterfly winged needles or plastic cannulae can be used. For short-term infusions, Butterfly winged needles are adequate and relatively easy to insert into even very small veins. A 23G needle is used most often, and is adequate for most purposes unless a large volume needs to be given rapidly. Smaller gauge needles, a short 25G or 27G, can be used in neonates, and are easier to stabilize as the needles are shorter. Now that plastic cannulae suitable for paediatric use are readily available, stainless steel Butterfly needles are used less often. Plastic cannulae have the advantage of lasting longer, as they do not cut out of the vein as readily. With practice, it is possible to insert them into the veins of even the tiniest preterm infants. A wide range of 22G plastic cannulae are available, e.g. Abbocath, Jelco, Vygon, Intraflow or Quick-Cath, and some are available in 24G, e.g. Quick-Cath, Wallace. Medicut cannulae are more difficult to insert as they are more rigid and are tapered.

Winged needles

For insertion of a winged needle, it is preferable to first splint the limb, otherwise a good infusion may be lost when the splint is applied. The needle and tubing of the winged needles should be filled with 0.9% saline to avoid the danger of air embolism. The syringe can then be removed or the connection between the tubing and the syringe loosened, so that as soon as the needle enters the vein blood will flow back into the tubing. The skin over the proposed site is cleaned with an alcohol swab. Depending on the site of the vein one may go through the skin and directly into the vein, or track a small distance beside the vein before entering it, or the vein may be entered at a Y junction which helps to fix it in position. To avoid piercing the vein stop advancing the needle as soon as blood flows back in the tubing. The needle can be stabilized with a strip of surgical tape across it and then flushed with a small amount of saline to remove any blood and prevent it clotting. This also tests the position of the needle; if there is resistance to flushing the syringe or swelling of the subcutaneous tissue the site is unsatisfactory. The skin will blanche if the vessel is an artery. The Butterfly can then be fixed more firmly and the tubing from the Butterfly and the giving set taped to the splint (Figure 8). A crepe bandage may then be applied leaving the

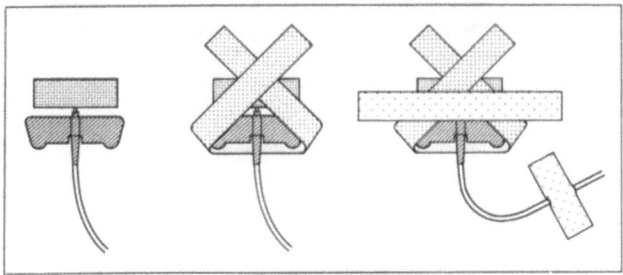

Figure 8   *A method of fixing a butterfly winged needle in infants*

area proximal to the tip of the needle exposed so that any extravasation of fluid will be recognized immediately. This is particularly important if hypertonic solutions, or solutions containing calcium or cytotoxic drugs are infused, or tissue damage (Figure 9a) with permanent scarring may occur (Figure 9b).

Scalp vein infusion

The most suitable veins are those in the midline over the frontal area (avoiding those overlying the anterior fontanelle), or those immediately in front or behind the ear. The temporal artery runs just anterior to the ear, and it is wise to palpate the chosen vessel to check that it is not an artery. The vessel selected should be of reasonable calibre and where the Butterfly will be able to rest satisfactorily on the scalp. The area should be shaved and then cleaned with isopropyl alcohol. Strips of surgical tape or plaster of paris should be prepared beforehand. All but the smallest infants need to be immobilized by wrapping them in a sheet or blanket. An assistant can hold the head steady and occlude the vein with a finger proximal to the site of insertion, or a tourniquet may be made with an elastic band around

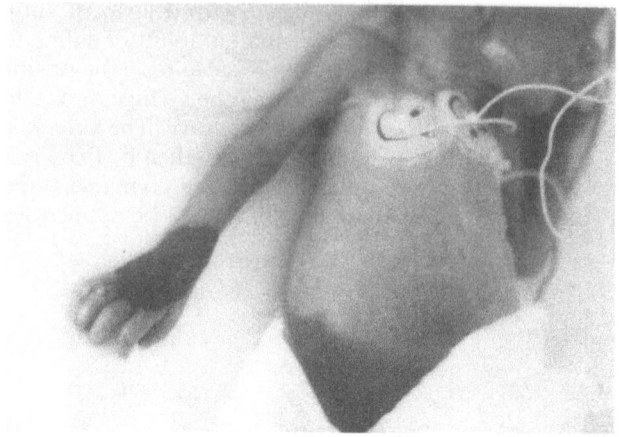

a

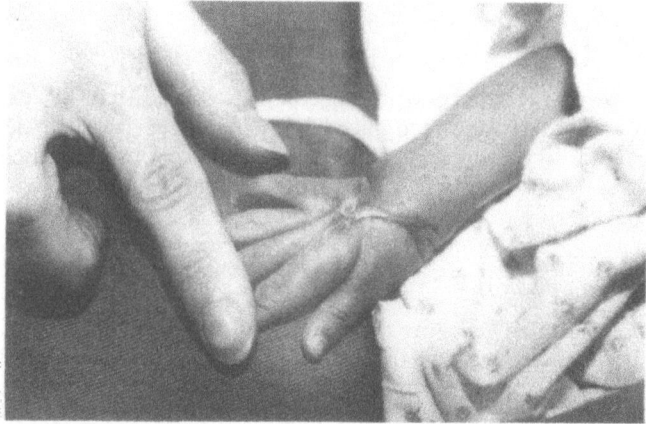

b

Figure 9   **a.** *Damage to the surrounding tissues after subcutaneous infiltration of an infusion of sodium bicarbonate.* **b.** *Subsequent scarring on the back of the hand*

the head. After insertion of the winged needle, it may be helpful to let it rest on some cotton wool to facilitate the flow. Plaster of Paris is useful to hold the Butterfly in position, but it is difficult to remove. If it is used, it is important that the tip of the needle is visible and not covered so that any extravasation of fluid is noted immediately (Figure 10). A loop of the Butterfly tubing needs to be taped to the

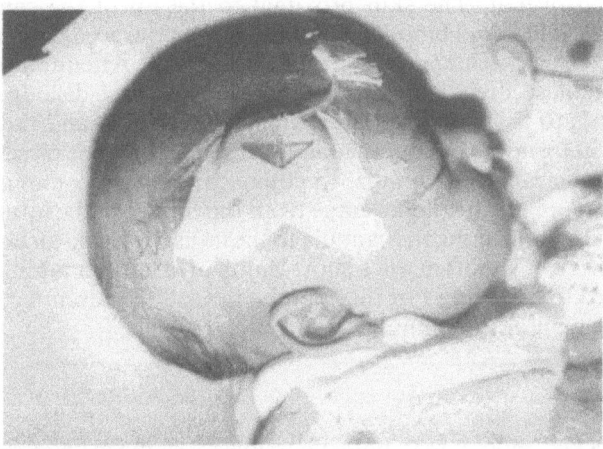

Figure 10   *Plaster of Paris used to fix a winged needle in a scalp vein infusion. The tip of the needle must be left clearly visible*

scalp so that the needle is not dislodged if the giving set is pulled. The larger gauge Butterfly needles (23G) are generally easier to insert as blood flows back into the tubing almost immediately the vein is entered, and this reduces the likelihood of advancing the needle too far. For very fine veins, a 25G or even 27G needle may be used. If necessary, the Butterfly can be protected by covering it with a plastic gallipot with two sections cut away, one for the needle to be visible, the other for the extension tubing, making sure that there are no sharp edges on the gallipot. If the solution infused may cause sloughing of the skin from subcutaneous leakage, it is best to avoid the frontal area of the scalp.

287

Cannulae

After cleaning the skin, local anaesthetic may be injected subcutaneously. It is helpful to first puncture the skin with a lancet before introducing the cannula. Entry of the vein is confirmed by flashback of the blood into the chamber. As the stylet projects beyond the end of the cannula, the needle should be held steady and the cannula advanced over it. The skin proximal to the tip of the cannula is compressed to avoid blood flowing back when the needle is removed, and the cannula is connected to the infusion set. Attention to fixing the cannula securely is important, or it may become dislodged. One method is to first pass the tape behind the cannula and then crisscross it in front of the cannula, and then apply another piece of tape at right angles to the cannula. In young children the cannula can be secured more firmly and leverage from the tubing to the infusion set avoided by connecting the cannula to the infusion set via an extension set with a 'T' (Abbot) or via a short length of extension tubing. These also need to be secured to the splint with tape to prevent accidental dislodgement of the cannula.

Cut-down

In a shocked child, it may not be possible to establish an intravenous infusion via a distal peripheral vein. It may be possible to insert a cannula into a vein in the antecubital fossa. The external jugular vein can sometimes be used in older children, but can be difficult in babies as their necks are short and chubby. The internal jugular vein can be used provided one is skilled in the technique. The femoral vein is another possible site.

Alternatively, a cut-down may be performed, using the long sapenous vein just anterior to the medial malleolus, or the cephalic or basilic veins in the antecubital fossa. Cut-downs are now used much less frequently, as it is almost always possible to establish an intravenous infusion percutaneously using a more central vein.

Central venous catheter

A central venous catheter may be needed as an emergency for treatment of shock and for measurement of the central venous pressure (CVP). Less urgently, they may be needed for intravenous nutrition or if an infusion cannot be established in any peripheral vein. The possible sites for percutaneous insertion of a central venous catheter are listed in Table 2. A venous cut-down can be used at some of these sites. Central venous catheters should not be inserted unless they are essential, as there are many possible complications (Table 3).

Table 2 Sites of percutaneous insertion of a central venous catheter

External jugular
Internal jugular: low approach
                   high approach, anterior or posterior
Supraclavicular
Infraclavicular
Antecubital fossa
Femoral vein

Table 3 Possible complications of central venous catheters

(a) *Insertion*
    Haematoma
    Pneumothorax
    Puncture of artery
    Damage to nerve and adjacent structures
    Cannulation of thoracic duct on the left side

(b) *Central venous line*
    Sepsis
    Thrombosis and emboli
    Damage or perforation of the heart or central vessels

The least hazardous site is the veins of the antecubital fossa. It is not always possible to advance the catheter centrally from this site but the success rate is higher if the basilic rather than the cephalic vein is used. The catheter may also be displaced when the arm is moved. This site is usually used in neonates for the percutaneous insertion of a central venous catheter for intravenous nutrition. Otherwise, a more reliable and quicker site is the internal jugular vein, using the anterior percutaneous approach, and this has the advantage that a larger gauge catheter can be inserted, which will give more reliable CVP readings. It is especially useful in an emergency situation, but it should only be done by someone experienced and competent in the procedure. Except in an emergency a general anaesthetic should be given.

All the equipment must be prepared and adequate assistance available. A 20-gauge cannula is suitable for neonates and an 18-gauge in infants. It is easier for a right-handed person to use the right jugular vein, and this has the advantage that the thoracic duct cannot be damaged. A towel is placed under the shoulders to extend the neck, and the head turned to face towards the left. The bed is tilted so that the patient is in a head downwards position which gives better filling of the vein and minimizes the risk of air embolism. The procedure must be done with full sterile precautions.

The carotid artery is palpated and retracted medially. At the anterior border of the sternomastoid muscle, at the level of the thyroid cartilage the needle is inserted at 60° to the skin and aligned towards the right nipple (Figure 11). The needle is advanced aspirating on a syringe until the vein is entered. The needle is then lowered to 40° to the skin and simultaneously advanced very slightly along the vein. Holding the needle and its tip stationary in the vein, the catheter is advanced over the needle or a catheter is threaded through

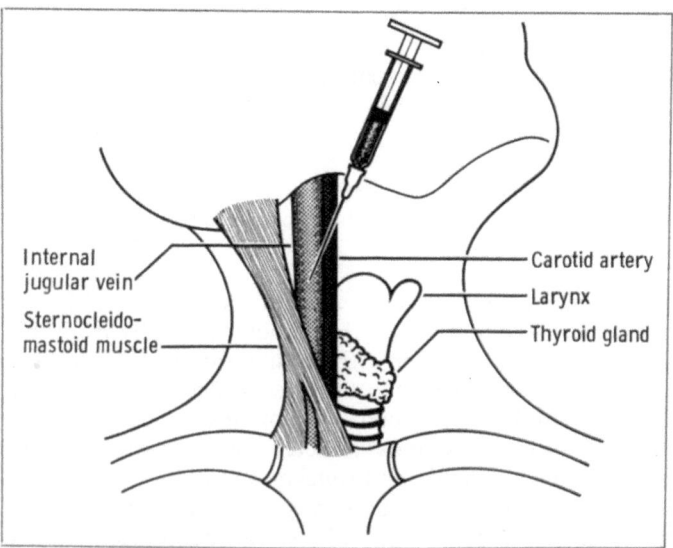

Figure 11 Site of insertion of a central venous catheter using the internal jugular vein

the needle, depending on the type of catheter used (Figure 12). The infusion is connected, and back flow along the line checked by lowering the bag with the infusion fluid below the level of table. If the back flow is slow, it may be necessary to insert a guide wire down the catheter to straighten out the tip or stop it impinging on the wall of the superior vena cava. The site of entry of the catheter can be covered with Betadine ointment. The catheter must be firmly secured, and its position checked radiographically.

When the catheter is used for intravenous nutrition a silicone catheter should be used, preferably tunnelled beneath the skin and meticulous attention paid to aseptic technique at insertion and during maintenance of the line.

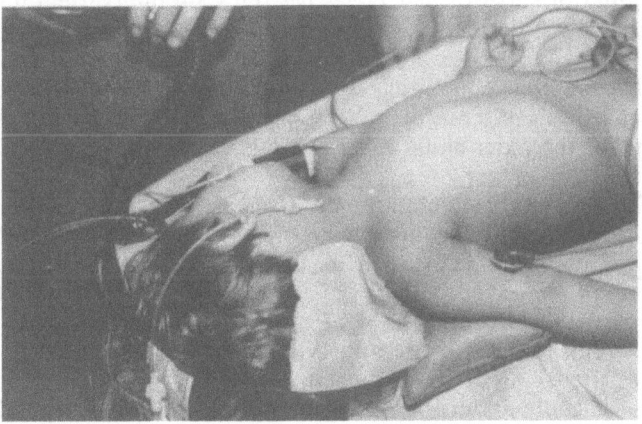

Figure 12   *A catheter (20G Abbocath) in the internal jugular vein inserted for central venous pressure monitoring. The catheter has not yet been secured*

Lumbar puncture

The incidence of meningitis is highest in the young. The presenting features are often non-specific and classical signs absent so that lumbar puncture is frequently needed in neonates and infants to exclude the diagnosis.

It is contraindicated if raised intracranial pressure is present on examination or suspected from the history as coning with herniation of the cerebellar tonsils through the foremen magnum may result. It should also be avoided if cord compression is suspected, or the skin over the lumbar area is infected.

It is best to first obtain a blood glucose and other blood samples. The assistance of an experienced nurse is essential. The lateral decubitus position is usually used, but holding neonates in a seated position may also be successful. In both situations good flexion of the neck and spine is essential, although the neck should not be flexed excessively, or the baby's airway may be occluded. Masks and gloves should be worn, and particular attention paid to sterilizing the skin. The spinal cord ends at the L1-2 level in adults and older children but somewhat lower in infants and neonates. Below the line joining both anterior superior iliac crests lies the L3-4 intervertebral space, and this space or the one below may be chosen. In neonates and infants local anaesthetic is often not used as it obscures the landmarks and if the lumbar puncture is done efficiently there seems to be little difference in the discomfort caused whether local anaesthetic is used or not. In the older child, local anaesthetic and sedation are often required.

A 22G disposable lumbar puncture needle with a stilette should be used in preference to a Butterfly needle, as it avoids the small risk of implantation dermoid cysts. After piercing the skin, ensure that the position of the patient and of the needle is optimal. The stilette can then be withdrawn and the needle slowly advanced until cerebrospinal fluid appears in the hub of the needle. The different tissue planes often cannot be appreciated in young children, and this method usually avoids obtaining blood stained cerebrospinal fluid from advancing the needle too far.

Suprapubic aspiration of urine

Obtaining satisfactory urine specimens for bacteriology in neonates and infants is difficult, and requires meticulous attention to detail. Urine may be collected as a clean catch mid-stream urine, with a urine collecting bag or by suprapubic aspiration of urine (SPA). An SPA is useful in an ill baby where an urgent screen for infection is being performed before starting antibiotics, if repeated results of bag specimens are equivocal, or to confirm the diagnosis of a urinary tract infection.

If the baby has had a wet nappy within the preceding 45 minutes, the procedure should preferably be delayed until a dull percussion note above the symphysis pubis suggests a full bladder. With an assistant holding the baby's legs in the frog position, the skin should be cleaned with povidone–iodine. From the start, it is best to have a urine container at the ready, as cleaning the skin and inserting the needle act as potent stimuli for babies to pass urine. It is sometimes recommended to prevent this in boys by gently squeezing the shaft of the penis. A 23G needle attached to a 5 or 10 ml syringe is used. The site of insertion is in the midline, about 1 cm above the symphysis pubis. This point usually lies just at the more proximal transverse skin crease. As the bladder is an abdominal organ at this age, the needle is angled at 20° to 40° to the perpendicular with the needle pointing cranially, and advanced 1–2 cms (Figure 13). Suction is

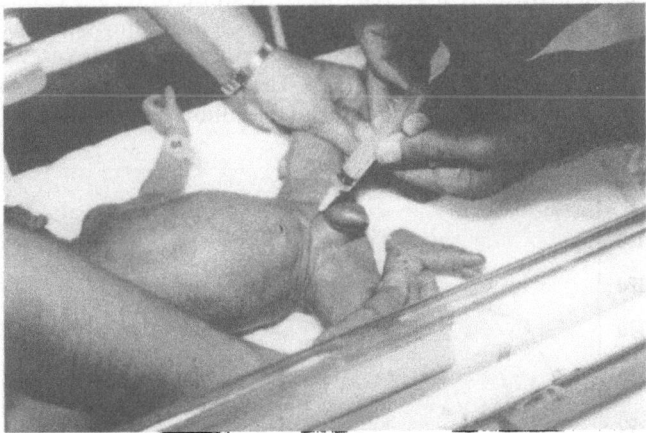

Figure 13 *Demonstration of the angle and site of insertion of the needle for a suprapubic aspiration of urine in a baby. As shown here, the procedure may act as a stimulus for the baby to pass urine!*

applied to the syringe whilst the needle is advanced so that it can be held steady as soon as the bladder is entered and urine is obtained, avoiding going on to puncture the bowel. If no urine is obtained, a further attempt can be made after an interval. Complications are haematuria, which is usually mild and transient, and occasionally the bowel is pierced, although this rarely causes any problems. The specimen must be taken to the bacteriology department and processed without delay. Any organisms on culture are indicative of a urinary tract infection, unless the bowel has been punctured.

Blood pressure

Measurement of the blood pressure should not be omitted when examining a child, and this is especially true if the child is very ill. It can be measured directly via an intra-arterial transducer, or usually indirectly with a sphygmomanometer. In children less than 5 years old, auscultation over the brachial artery with a stethoscope may be difficult and is less accurate than using a Doppler ultrasound machine. It is important to use the right size sphygmomanometer cuff. The cuffbladder must completely encircle the arm, and its width needs to be at least two-thirds of the length of the upper arm. Too small a cuff will result in artificially high readings. Meaningful results cannot be obtained if the baby or toddler is crying. Determining the diastolic blood pressure accurately with a sphygmomanometer is often difficult or impossible in young children. The chart showing the normal range of systolic blood pressure during childhood is shown in Figure 14.

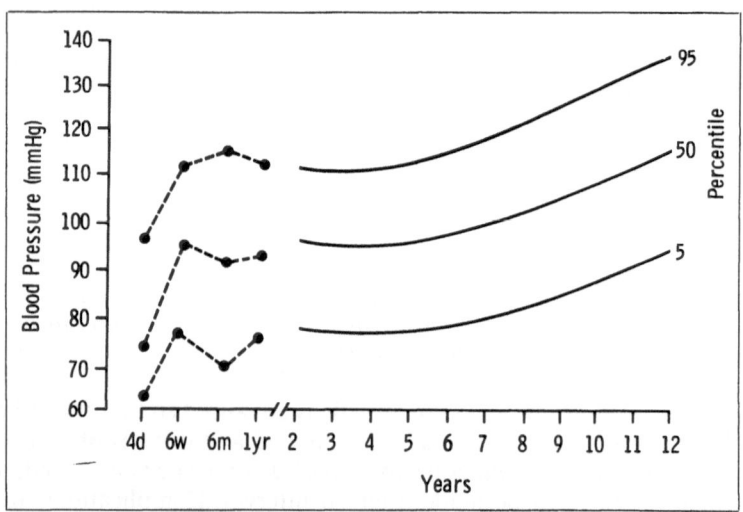

Figure 14   *Systolic blood pressure in normal infants and children, measured when awake. (de Swiet et al., 1980). Data from Brompton study and Task Force for Blood Pressure in Children (1977), reproduced with permission of the authors and publishers*

References

de Swiet, M., Fayers, P. and Shinebourne, E.A. (1980), *Pediatrics*, **65**, 5, 1028-35.
Report on the Task Force on Blood Pressure Control in Children (1977), *Pediatrics*, **59**, (Suppl).
Shaw, J. (1968), *Lancet*, **2**, 389-390.

Further reading

Two approaches to cannulation of a child's internal jugular vein (1979), *Anesthesiology*, **50**, 371.

Appendix

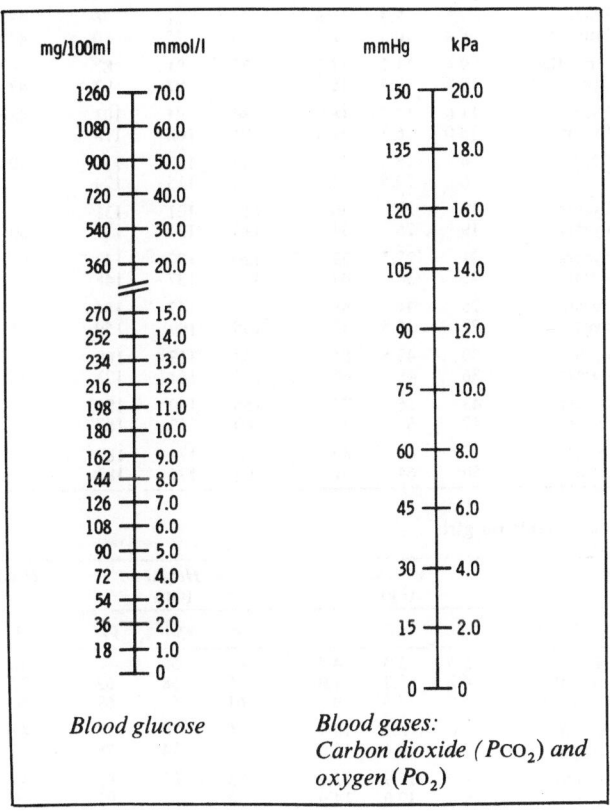

mg/100ml	mmol/l		mmHg	kPa
1260	70.0		150	20.0
1080	60.0			
900	50.0		135	18.0
720	40.0			
540	30.0		120	16.0
360	20.0		105	14.0
270	15.0			
252	14.0		90	12.0
234	13.0			
216	12.0		75	10.0
198	11.0			
180	10.0			
162	9.0		60	8.0
144	8.0			
126	7.0		45	6.0
108	6.0			
90	5.0			
72	4.0		30	4.0
54	3.0			
36	2.0		15	2.0
18	1.0			
	0		0	0

Blood glucose

Blood gases:
Carbon dioxide (P_{CO_2}) and
oxygen (P_{O_2})

SI unit conversions

Centile table for boys

Age	Weight (kg)			Height (cm)			Head circumference (cm)		
Centile	3	50	97	3	50	97	3	50	97
Birth	2.5	3.5	4.4	—	50	—	33	35	38
3 months	4.4	5.7	7.2	55	60	65	38	41	43
6 months	6.2	7.8	9.8	62	66.5	71	41	44	46
9 months	7.6	9.3	11.6	66.5	71	76	43	46	47
12 months	8.4	10.3	12.8	70	75	80	44	47	49
18 months	9.4	11.7	14.2	75	81	87	46	49	51
2 years	10.2	12.7	15.5	80	87	93	47	50	52
3 years	11.6	14.7	18.0	86	94	101	48	50	53
4 years	13.0	16.7	20.4	94	102	110			
5 years	14.4	18.5	23.2	99	108	117	49	51	54
6 years	16	20.5	26.5	105	115	124			
7 years	17	23	30	110	121	131			
8 years	19	25	34	115	126	137	50	52	55
9 years	21	27.5	39	120	132	143			
10 years	23	30	44	125	137	148			
11 years	25	34	48	130	142	154			
12 years	27	36.5	53	135	147	159	51	54	56
13 years	30	40.5	64	138	153	168			
14 years	36	48	66	148	161	173	53	56	58
15 years	43	56	74	156	169	181			
16 years	47	60	78	160	172	187			
17 years	49	62	80	162	174	187			
18 years	50	64	81	162	175	187			

Centile table for girls

Age	Weight (kg)			Height (cm)			Head circumference (cm)		
Centile	3	50	97	3	50	97	3	50	97
Birth	2.5	3.5	4.4	—	50	—	32	35	37
3 months	4.2	5.2	7.0	55	58	62	37	40	43
6 months	5.9	7.3	9.4	61	65	69	40	43	45
9 months	7.0	8.7	10.9	65	70	74	42	44	47
12 months	7.6	9.6	12.0	69	74	78	43	46	48
18 months	8.8	10.9	13.6	75	80	85	45	47	50
2 years	9.6	12.0	14.9	79	85	91	46	48	51
3 years	11.2	14.4	17.6	86	93	100	47	49	52
4 years	13	16	20	92	100	109			
5 years	15	18	23	98	107	116	48	50	53
6 years	16	20	27	104	114	123			
7 years	18	23	30	109	119	130			
8 years	19	25	35	114	125	136	50	52	54
9 years	21	28	40	120	130	142			
10 years	23	31	45	125	136	147			
11 years	25	34	50	130	142	153			
12 years	29	40	58	138	149	161	51	53	56
13 years	37	47	66	145	157	168			
14 years	42	53	71	149	160	172	52	54	57
15 years	44	55	74	150	162	173			
16 years	45	56	75	151	162	174			
17 years	46	56	75	—	—	—			
18 years	46	57	75	—	—	—			

Weight and height centiles adapted from Tanner, J. M., Whitehouse, R. H. and Takaishi, M. (1966). *Arch. Dis. Child.*, **41**, 454.
Head circumference centiles adapted from Westrop, C. K. and Barber, C. R. (1956). *J. Neurol. Neurosurg. Psychiatr.*, **19**, 52.

Drug doses for children

A list follows of the commonly prescribed drugs in acute paediatrics. The dose stated is for **each individual dose prescribed** and the recommended number of times it is given per 24 hours has been stated. It is not the total daily dosage.

Drug doses in children can be estimated according to age, body weight or surface area. Calculations based on surface area are generally agreed to be the most reliable way to estimate dosage for a child. A nomogram is needed to calculate the surface area. It is easier in practice to express doses as a percentage of the adult dose. Table 1 shows a comparison of the dose expressed as a percentage of the adult level based on the surface area when applied to a child of average size.

Doses may also be expressed in terms of weight but a uniform scheme suitable for children of all ages cannot be formulated on this basis. In addition the dose for an obese child may be overestimated as fat plays little part in drug metabolism. These factors are automatically recognized when using the percentage method which compensates for the relatively larger surface area of children in relation to their weight and so this method of dose estimation has been adopted. For children under one year the dose has been shown on a mg/kg basis because of the rapid growth in this period. It actually results in a slight underdosage in the first few months of life. In view of the very different metabolism and excretion of drugs in neonates a separate list has been made for the neonatal period.

Full details of the indications for use of the various drugs and their side effects can be found in the *British National Formulary* and the *Paediatric Prescriber* by P. Catzel and R. Olver (Blackwell Scientific Publications, Oxford, 1981).

Table 1 Doses for different ages as percent of adult dose

Adult	100%
7 years	50%
3 years	33%
1 year	approx 25%

299

Drug doses

Drug	Route	Times daily	Dosage per dose given					Remarks
			0–2 weeks	2 weeks–1 year	1 year	7 years	Adult	
Adrenaline (epinephrine) 1:1000	s.c.	Single dose	—0.01 ml/kg—		0.125 ml	0.25 ml	0.5 ml	For asthma, anaphylaxis. Repeat after 15 min × 2 if necessary.
1:10 000	i.v. Down ET tube Intracardiac	Single dose	—0.01 ml/kg—		1 ml	2.5 ml	5 ml	For cardiac arrest, life threatening anaphylaxis. May produce arrythmias.
	Continuous infusion		—0.5–1.5 μg kg^{-1} min^{-1}—					For profound hypotension. Increase dose according to response.
Allopurinol (Zyloric)	oral	3	—	5 mg/kg	50 mg	100 mg	200 mg	For prevention of uric acid nephropathy in malignant disease.
Amikacin (Amikin)	i.m. i.v.	2	See Table 2	—7.5 mg/kg—			7.5 mg/kg	Side-effects—as Gentamicin.
Aminophylline	i.v.		Loading dose 6.2 mg/kg then 4.4 mg kg^{-1} (24 h)$^{-1}$ by continuous infusion	Loading dose: 5–6 mg/kg, over 20 min then by continuous infusion: 1 mg kg^{-1} h^{-1} if <9 y, or: 0.7 mg kg^{-1} h^{-1} if >9 y				For status asthmaticus. Monitor levels if necessary. Arrythmias, convulsions may occur. Apnoea in preterm infants.

Drug	Route	Freq						Notes
Aminophylline, slow release (Phyllocontin)	oral	2	—	——10–14 mg/kg——			225–450 mg	For asthma. Monitor levels. Tablets 225, 100 mg.
Amoxycillin (Amoxil)	oral	3	——62.5 mg——		125 mg	250 mg	500 mg	Syrup 125 mg/5 ml.
Ampicillin (Penbritin)	i.v. i.m.	4	See Table 2	12.5–25 mg/kg	125 mg	250 mg	500 mg	Meningitis: 400 mg kg^{-1} (24 h)$^{-1}$.
	oral	4	——62.5 mg——		125 mg	250 mg	500 mg	Syrup 125 mg/5 ml.
	i.v. i.m.	4	See Table 2	12.5–25 mg/kg	125 mg	250 mg	500 mg	Meningitis: 400 mg kg^{-1} (24 h)$^{-1}$.
Aspirin, soluble	oral	3 or 4	Not suitable—use paracetamol		100 mg	300 mg	600 mg	As antipyretic, analgesia. Soluble tablets 300 mg. Paediatric 75 mg. Antirheumatic: 100 mg kg^{-1} (24 h)$^{-1}$ divided 4–6 hourly and measure salicylate level.
Atropine	i.v.	Single dose	—0.01–0.03 mg/kg—		0.15 mg	0.3 mg	0.6 mg	For cardiac arrest, bradycardia.
Azlocillin (Securopen)	i.v.	4	See Table 2	50–100 mg/kg	500 mg	1 g	2 g	Double dose in severe infections. May cause hypokalaemia.
Bendro-fluazide	oral	Once	——0.125 mg/kg——		1.25 mg	2.5 mg	5 mg	Potassium supplement required.
Calcium chloride (10%)	i.v.	Single	——0.1 ml/kg——		1.2 ml	2.5 ml	5 ml	For cardiac arrest, asystole. Inject slowly under ECG control. Very irritant if infusion tissues.
Calcium gluconate (10%)	i.v.	Single	——3 ml/kg——		3.5 ml	7.5 ml	15 ml	For cardiac arrest, asystole.
	i.v.	Single	0.2 ml/kg		—			Neonatal tetany. Inject slowly. May cause bradycardia.

Drug	Route	Times daily	Dosage per dose given					Remarks
			0–2 weeks	2 weeks–1 year	1 year	7 years	Adult	
Carbamazepine (Tegretol)	oral	2 or 3	–	10 mg/kg	100 mg	200 mg	400 mg	
Carbenicillin (Pyopen)	i.v.	4	See Table 2	50–100 mg/kg	500 mg	1 g	2 g	Dose may be doubled in severe infections. May cause hypokalaemia.
Cefuroxime (Zinacef)	i.m. or i.v.	3	See Table 2	20 mg/kg	200 mg	375 mg	750 mg	
Cephazolin (Kefzol)	i.m. or i.v.	4	–	12.5–25 mg/kg	125 mg	250 mg	500 mg	
Cephalexin (Ceporex, Keflex)	oral	4	——— 12 mg/kg ———		125 mg	250 mg	500 mg	
Cephradine (Velosef)	oral	4	——— 12 mg/kg ———		125 mg	250 mg	500 mg	
	i.m. or i.v.	4	See Table 2	12.5–25 mg/kg	125 mg	250 mg	500 mg	
Charcoal activated (Medicoal)	oral	Single	–	——— 0.5–1 g/kg with water ———			10–50 g in 50 ml water	Acute poisoning.
Chloral hydrate	oral	Single	——— 30 mg/kg ———		300 mg	500 mg	1.0 g	Single hypnotic dose. Elixir 200 mg/5 ml, 500 mg/5 ml.
Chloramphenicol (Chloromycetin)	oral i.v.	4	See Table 2	12.5 mg/kg	——— 12.5–25 mg/kg ———		1.0 g	May cause aplastic anaemia.

Drug	Route	Frequency	(mg/kg)				Notes
Chlorothiazide (Saluric)	oral	2	——10 mg/kg——	125 mg	250 mg	500 mg	Potassium supplement needed.
Chloroquine (as base) (Nivaquine)	oral	Initial dose:	15 mg/kg	150 mg	300 mg	600 mg	For benign tertian malaria. Follow with Primaquine for 14 days. For *P. falciparum* from chloroquine resistant area use quinine or Fansidar (pyrimethamine and sulfadoxine)
		then given 6 h later:	7.5 mg/kg	75 mg	150 mg	300 mg	
		then dose given 12-hourly for 2 days:	3.75 mg/kg	37.5 mg	75 mg	150 mg	
Chlorpheniramine (Piriton)	oral i.v.	3 or 4 Single	— 0.25 mg/kg	1 mg 2.5 mg	2 mg 5 mg	4 mg 10 mg	Acute anaphylaxis
Choline theophyllinate (Choledyl)	oral	3	5 mg/kg	50 mg	100 mg	200 mg	Monitor levels. Tablets 100 mg and 200 mg. Syrup 62.5 mg/5 ml.
Cimetidine (Tagamet)	oral	4	——5–10 mg/kg——		100 mg tds and 200 mg at night	200 mg tds and 400 mg at night	Tablets 200 mg. Syrup 200 mg/5 ml.
	i.v. (over 2 hours)	4	——4 mg/kg——		100 mg	200 mg	
Clonazepam (Rivotril)	oral maintenance dose	4	—	0.25 mg	0.5 mg	1 mg	2 mg	Anticonvulsant. May cause drowsiness and increased salivation. Start with dose stated once a day, and gradually increase.

Drug	Route	Times daily	Dosage per dose given					Remarks
			0–2 weeks	2 weeks– 1 year	1 year	7 years	Adult	
Co-trimoxazole (Septrin, Bactrim)	oral	2	See Table 2	24 mg/kg	240 mg	480 mg	960 mg	Dose given in terms of total of Trimethoprin 1 part and Sulphamethoxazole 5 parts. Tablets: 960, 480, 120 mg. Suspension: 480 mg/ 5 ml. Paediatric syrup 240 mg/5 ml.
	i.v.	Prophy-lactic at night	See Table 2	12 mg/kg	120 mg	240 mg	480 mg	
Desferrioxamine (Desferal)	i.m. and i.v.	Single	—	20 mg/kg given i.m. immediately. If necessary, then i.v. 80 mg/kg over 24 hours. Rate not to exceed 15 mg/kg.				For severe iron poisoning. May cause hypotension.
Dexamethasone (Decadron, Oradexon)	i.v.	4	——0.1 mg/kg——		1 mg	2 mg	4 mg	For cerebral oedema. May initially give double this dose. In Gram-negative shock, up to 10 times stated dose.
Dextrose, 50%	i.v.	Single	—————— up to 4 ml/kg (2 g/kg)——————					For hypoglycaemia. Dilute before injection.
Diazepam (Valium, Diazemuls)	i.v. slowly	Single	——0.25 mg/kg——		2.5 mg	5 mg	10 mg	As anticonvulsant or for sedation. May repeat in 15 min if necessary. May cause respiratory depression. Injection: 5 mg/ ml.
Diazoxide (Eudemine)	i.v.	Up to 4	—		3–5 mg/kg		300 mg	For severe hypertension. May cause hypotension. Inject rapidly.
Dichloral-phenazone (Welldorm)	oral	Once	——22.5 mg/kg——		225 mg	650 mg	1.3 g	For sedation. Tablets 650 mg. Elixir 225 mg/5 ml.
Dicyclomine (Merbentyl)	oral	4	——5 mg——		—	—	—	For three month colic. Give 15 min before feed. Syrup 10 mg/5 ml.
Digoxin (Lanoxin)			see page 215					

Drug	Route	Frequency					Comments
Disopyramide (Norpace, Rhythmodan)	i.v.	Single	2 mg/kg to max of 150 mg, slowly, then 0.4 mg kg⁻¹ h⁻¹ by continuous infusion				For ventricular arrhythmias, paroxysmal supraventricular tachycardia.
Dioctyl sodium sulphosuccinate (Dioctyl-Medo)	oral	3	—	12.5-25 mg	20 mg	40 mg	
Dopamine (Intropin)	i.v.	Single	5–20 µg kg⁻¹ min⁻¹. Adjust dose according to response				Inotropic agent for hypotension and poor cardiac output. Correct hypovolaemia first. May cause arrhythmias.
Dobutamine hydrochloride (Dobutrax)	i.v.	Single	2.5–10 µg kg⁻¹ min⁻¹. Adjust dose according to response				Inotropic agent.
Droperidol (Droleptan)	i.v. i.m. oral	Single	0.1 mg/kg	1.25 mg	2.5 mg	5 mg	For sedation or premedication. Tablets 2.5 mg, 10 mg.
Erythromycin (Erythrocin, Erythroped, Ilosone)	oral	4	12 mg/kg	125 mg	250 mg	500 mg	
Ethambutol (Myambutol)	oral	Once	12–25 mg/kg				May cause ocular toxicity.
Ethosuximide (Zarontin, Emeside)	oral	Once	—	12 mg/kg (up to 50 mg/kg)	250 mg (max. 1 g)	500 mg (max. 2 g)	Initial dose. Increase by 250 mg every 4–7 days according to response, to maximum dose.
Ferrous sulphate	oral	3	6 mg/kg	60 mg	120 mg	200 mg	Treatment of iron deficiency anaemia. Tablets 200 mg and 300 mg. Paediatric mixture 60 mg/5 ml.

Drug	Route	Times daily	Dosage per dose given					Remarks
			0–2 weeks	2 weeks– 1 year	1 year	7 years	Adult	
Flucloxacillin (Floxapen) and cloxacillin (Orbenin)	oral i.m. or i.v.	4	See Table 2	62.5 mg	125 mg	250 mg	500 mg	Better oral absorption with flucloxacillin. Syrup 125 mg/5 ml.
Folic acid	oral	Once	—	0.25 mg/kg	2.5 mg	5 mg	10 mg	Tablets 0.1 mg and 5 mg.
Frusemide (Lasix)	oral	Once	——2 mg/kg——		20 mg	40 mg	80 mg	Needs K supplements unless given with spironolactone. Paediatric mixture 1 mg/ml.
	i.m. i.v.	Single	——1 mg/kg——		10 mg	20 mg	40 mg	Double the dose if necessary.
Fusidic acid (Fucidin)	oral	4	—	12.5 mg/kg as fusidic acid		250 mg as sodium fusidate	500 mg as sodium fusidate	Fusidic acid suspension 250 mg/5 ml. Capsules, sodium fusidate 250 mg.
	i.v.	3	—	12.5 mg/kg	125 mg	250 mg	500 mg	Given as a continuous infusion.
Gentamicin (Genticin, Cidomycin)	i.m. i.v.	3	See Table 2	————2 mg/kg————				May be ototoxic and nephrotoxic. Monitor serum levels. Increase time between doses in renal failure. Do not combine with carbenicillin in same infusion.
Glucagon	i.m. i.v.	Single	25–100 µg/kg——		0.25 mg	0.5 mg	1 mg	For hypoglycaemia.
Glycerol	oral	4	————1 g/kg————					Used in North America for cerebral oedema.
Hydralazine (Apresoline)	i.v. i.m.	4	————0.2–0.4 mg/kg————					For severe hypertension.

Drug	Route	Doses						Notes
Hydrocortisone	i.v.	4–6	—	5 mg/kg	50 mg	100 mg	200 mg	For status asthmaticus. For Gram-negative shock, initial dose up to 5 times dose stated. Injection: 100 mg as sodium succinate.
Indomethacin (Indocid)	oral	Single	0.2 mg/kg	—	—	—	—	In neonates, to close a patent ductus arteriosus. Repeat × 2, 8 hourly if necessary.
Ipecacuanha	oral	Single	—	10 ml	15 ml	15 ml	30 ml	Paediatric ipecacuanha—emetic mixture. Repeat after 20 min if necessary.
Ipratropium (Atrovent)	nebulized	3	—	—	0.1–0.5 mg in 2 ml sterile water			For status asthmaticus in children over 3 y.
Isoniazid	oral	Once	7.5 mg/kg	7.5 mg/kg	75 mg	150 mg	300 mg	
Isoprenaline (Isoproterenol; Isuprel)	i.v.	Once	0.1–$0.5\ \mu g\ kg^{-1}\ min^{-1}$ by continuous infusion. Adjust dose according to the response					Inotropic agent for bradycardia, hypotension and poor cardiac output.
Lactulose (Duphalac, Gafinar)	oral	Once	—	5 ml	10 ml	20 ml	30 ml	Dose of elixir, containing lactulose 3.35 g/5 ml.
Lignocaine (Xylocard)	i.v.	Once	Bolus of 1 mg/kg, repeat after 5 min if necessary, then 10–$50\ \mu g\ kg^{-1}\ min^{-1}$ by continuous infusion					For ventricular tachycardia.
Magnesium sulphate (50%)	i.m. i.v.	Single	0.1 mg/kg	—	—	—	—	For neonatal hypomagnesaemia. Give i.v. injection slowly.
Mannitol (20%)	i.v. over 20 min	Single	0.5–1 g/kg					For cerebral oedema. Repeat as indicated. May cause circulatory overload. Monitor osmolality.

Drug	Route	Times daily	Dosage per dose given					Remarks
			0–2 weeks	2 weeks–1 year	1 year	7 years	Adult	
Methicillin (Celbenin)	i.m. i.v.	4	See Table 2	25 mg/kg	250 mg	500 mg	1 g	Increase according to response, up to 3 times stated dose.
Methyldopa (Aldomet, Copamet, Medomet)	oral	3	—	6 mg/kg	62.5 mg	125 mg	250 mg	
Metoclopramide (Maxolon, Primperan)	oral i.m. i.v.	3 Single Single	—	0.1 mg/kg	1 mg	5 mg	10 mg	Syrup 5 mg/5 ml. Paediatric liquid 1 mg/ml. Tablets 10 mg.
Metronidazole (Flagyl)	oral rectal i.v.	3 3 3		7.5 mg/kg 7.5 mg/kg 7.5 mg/kg			400 mg 1 g 500 mg	For anaerobic infections.
Morphine sulphate	i.m. i.v.	Single		0.2 mg/kg	2.5 mg	5 mg	10 mg	May cause respiratory depression, especially in young children.
Nalidixic acid (Negram)	oral	4		—	250 mg	500 mg	1 g	Suspension 300 mg/5 ml. For prophylaxis, give only twice daily.
Naloxone HCl (Narcon)	i.m. i.v.	Single	0.01 mg/kg		0.1 mg	0.2 mg	0.4 mg	Narcotic overdosage. Repeat in 2 min if necessary. Injection 400 µg/ml. Neonatal 20 µg/ml.
Neomycin sulphate (Nivemycin)	oral	4	25 mg/kg		250 mg	500 mg	1 g	
Nitrofurantoin (Furadantin)	oral	4	Avoid	2.5 mg/kg	25 mg	50 mg	100 mg	Tablets 50 mg, 100 mg. Suspension 25 mg/5 ml. For prophylaxis, give twice daily. Contraindicated in infants <1 month old.

Drug	Route	Doses per day	Dose/kg					Notes
Nystatin (Nystan)	oral	4	For oral thrush, 100000 units					Suspension 100000 units/ml.
Papaveretum (Omnopon)	oral, i.m., i.v.	Single	200 µg/kg	—	2.5–5 mg	5–10 mg	10–20 mg	For sedation, analgesia, premedication. Dose of Omnopon-Scopolamine is 0.03 ml/kg i.m. (papaveretum 20 mg and hyoscine 400 µg/ml) 1 hour before operation.
Paracetamol (Acetaminophen Panadol, Calpol, Tylenol (USA))	oral	4–6	24 mg/kg	—	240 mg	500 mg	1 g	Tablets 500 mg, suspension (Calpol) 120 mg/5 ml.
Paraldehyde	i.m.	Single dose	0.15 ml/kg	1 ml	5 ml		10 ml	To avoid sterile abscesses, give deep i.m. Repeat in 15–30 min if necessary.
	rectal	Single dose	0.3 ml/kg					Mix with equal volume of mineral oil.
Penicillin G (benzyl penicillin, Crystapen)	i.m., i.v.	4	See Table 2 / 15 mg/kg	150 mg	300 mg	600 mg		Increase dose and frequency in severe infections.
Penicillin, prolonged action (benethamine penicillin, Triplopen)	i.m.	Every 2–3 days		¼ vial	½ vial	1 vial		One vial contains benethamine penicillin 475 mg, procaine penicillin 250 mg, benzylpenicillin 300 mg.
Penicillin V (phenoxymethyl penicillin) (Crystapen V, V-Cil-K etc).	oral	4	62.5 mg	125 mg	250 mg	500 mg		Syrup 125 mg, 250 mg/5 ml.

Drug	Route	Times daily	Dosage per dose given					Remarks
			0-2 weeks	2 weeks-1 year	1 year	7 years	Adult	
Pethidine	i.m.	Single	——1-2 mg/kg——			25-50 mg	50-100 mg	For analgesia, sedation, premedication 1 hour before operation.
Phenobarbitone	oral	Once	——4-6 mg/kg——			60-120 mg	60-360 mg	As an anticonvulsant. May cause behaviour disturbance in some children.
	i.v.	Single	——5-10 mg/kg——				—	Status epilepticus. May cause respiratory depression. Repeat after 20 min if necessary.
Phenytoin (Epanutin)	oral	2	—	3 mg/kg	30 mg	50 mg	100 mg	Maintenance anticonvulsant therapy. Side effects include gum hypertrophy, ataxia and liver damage. Tablets 50, 100 mg. Suspension 30 mg/5 ml.
	i.v. (slow)		——————15-20 mg/kg——————				—	Status epilepticus. May cause hypotension and cardiac dysrhythmias.
Phytomenadione (Vit K, Konakion)	oral i.m. i.v.	Single	1 mg	1 mg	3 mg	5 mg	10 mg	
Potassium supplements	oral	Once	——————1-2 mmol K^+ kg^{-1} $(24 h)^{-1}$——————					Starting dose in diuretic therapy. Base dose on clinical requirements and plasma K. Give as potassium chloride, or potassium gluconate, or effervescent potassium (potassium bicarbonate).
Prednisolone	oral	Once	——2 mg kg^{-1} $(24 h)^{-1}$ or 60 mg m^{-2} $(24 h)^{-1}$——					For induction of remission in nephrotic syndrome. Minimum dose 25 mg/24 h, max 80 mg/24 h.
Primaquine	oral	Once	—	375 μg/kg	3.75 mg	7.5 mg	15 mg	For eradication of benign tertian malaria. Give for 14 days after treatment with chloroquine. Test for G6PD deficiency. Tablets only, 7.5 mg.

Drug	Route	Freq						Comments
Promethazine HCl (Phenergan)	oral	3	—	0.5 mg/kg	5 mg	10 mg	25 mg	For use as an antihistamine. For single sedative dose the stated dose can be doubled.
Propranolol (Inderal)	oral	3	—— 0.2–0.3 mg/kg. Max dose 20 mg ——				—	For arrhythmias.
	i.v.	Single	—— 0.1–0.15 mg/kg. Max single dose 10 mg ——				—	For arrhythmias, cyanotic attacks in tetralogy of Fallot. Repeat in 6 hours if necessary.
Prostaglandin E$_1$ and E$_2$	i.v.	Single	0.05–1 μg kg^{-1} min^{-1} as an infusion	—	—	—	—	1.5 mg prostaglandin in 500 ml dextrose. Give via a syringe pump.
Rifampicin (Rifadin, Rimactane)	oral	Once	—	15 mg/kg	150 mg	300 mg	600 mg	May cause urine, saliva to go red. In prophylaxis for meningococcal or *H. influenzae* contacts, 2–4 days only. Capsules, 150, 300 mg. Suspension 100 mg/5 ml.
Salbutamol (Ventolin)	oral	3–4	—	0.1 mg/kg	1 mg	2 mg	4 mg	Tablets 2 mg, 4 mg, 8 mg (long-acting). Syrup 2 mg/5 ml.
	inhalation (powder)	4	—	—	—	200 μg	200–400 μg	Rotacaps 200, 400 μg with Rotahaler.
	nebulizer	4–8	—	0.05 ml/kg	0.5 ml	1 ml	2 ml	In status asthmaticus. Respirator solution 0.5% made up to 2 ml with normal saline.
	i.v.	—	—	5–7 μg kg^{-1} h^{-1} given hourly or by continuous infusion	—	—	250 μg every 4 h or 200–1200 μg/h by continuous infusion	In status asthmaticus.

Drug	Route	Times daily	Dosage per dose given					Remarks
			0–2 weeks	2 weeks–1 year	1 year	7 years	Adult	
Sodium bicarbonate	i.v.	—	—————— 1–2 mmol/kg ——————					For cardiac arrest. After initial dose, according to blood gases.
Sodium cromoglycate (Intal)	inhaled	4	—	—	—	———— 1–2 puffs ————		Inhaler 20 mg per puff. For young children 10–20 mg by nebulizer (nebulizer solution 10 mg/ml).
Sodium nitroprusside (Nipride)	i.v.	Single	—0.5 μg kg^{-1} min^{-1} initially, adjust according to response to 5 μg kg^{-1} min^{-1} —					For severe hypertension. Potent vasodilator. Monitor blood pressure.
Sodium valproate (Epilim; Valproic acid, Depakene in USA)	oral	3	—	———7–10 mg/kg———		100–200 mg	200–400 mg	Start with lower dose, increase if necessary every 3 days to higher dose. Maximum adult dose is 2.6 g daily. For prophylaxis of febrile convulsions, can use 20–30 mg kg^{-1} (24 h)$^{-1}$, given twice a day. Increases phenobarbitone levels. Tablets 200 mg. Syrup 200 mg/5 ml.
Spironolactone (Aldactone, Spiroctan)	oral	2–4	———— 0.625 mg/kg ————		6.25 mg	12.5 mg	25 mg	Counteracts K loss of other diuretics. Contraindicated in acute renal failure. Tablets 25 mg (crushable).
Terbutaline (Bricanyl)	oral	3	—	0.15 mg/kg	1.5 mg	3 mg	5 mg	Reduce dose if there is tremor, nervousness, nausea. For status asthmaticus.
	s.c. slow i.v.	2–4	—	5–10 μg/kg	50–100 μg	100–200 μg	250–500 μg	
	spacer inhaler	3–4	—	—	—	250 μg (1 puff)	250–500 μg (1–2 puffs)	
	nebulizer	4	—	0.2 mg/kg	2 mg	5 mg	10 mg	For status asthmaticus. Nebulizer solution 10 mg/ml. Make up to 2 ml with normal saline.

Drug	Route	Frequency	Dose					Comments
Theophylline, slow release (Rona-Slophyllin)	oral	2	—		—12 mg/kg—		125–250 mg	250–500 mg	Dose of Rona-Slophyllin (Gyrocaps 60, 125, 250 mg). Pellets can be removed from capsule and swallowed (but not chewed).
Thyroxine (Eltroxin)	oral	Once		—12.5 µg—	25 µg	50 µg	100 µg	Initial dose, adjust according to response. Tablets 25, 50, 100 µg.
Trimeprazine tartrate (Vallergan)	oral	Single		—2–4 mg/kg—				For sedation, premedication 1–2 hours beforehand.
		3–4	—	0.25 mg/kg	2.5 mg	5 mg	10 mg	For pruritus. Syrup 7.5 mg/5 ml. Syrup forte 30 mg/5 ml.
Tobramycin (Nebcin)	i.v. i.m.	3	See Table 2	—2 mg/kg—			1–2 mg/kg	Side-effects similar to Gentamicin. Measure serum levels.
Tolazoline HCl (Priscol)	i.v.	—	Bolus of 2 mg/kg then 1–2 mg kg^{-1} h^{-1} by infusion	—	—	—		In neonates for pulmonary hypertension especially in persistent fetal circulation. Monitor blood pressure. May cause GI haemorrhage.
Verapamil (Cordilox) *Dosage per dose given*	i.v. slow			—0.05–1.5 mg/kg—		2.5 mg	5 mg	Supraventricular dysrhythmias. Repeat after 5–10 min if necessary.

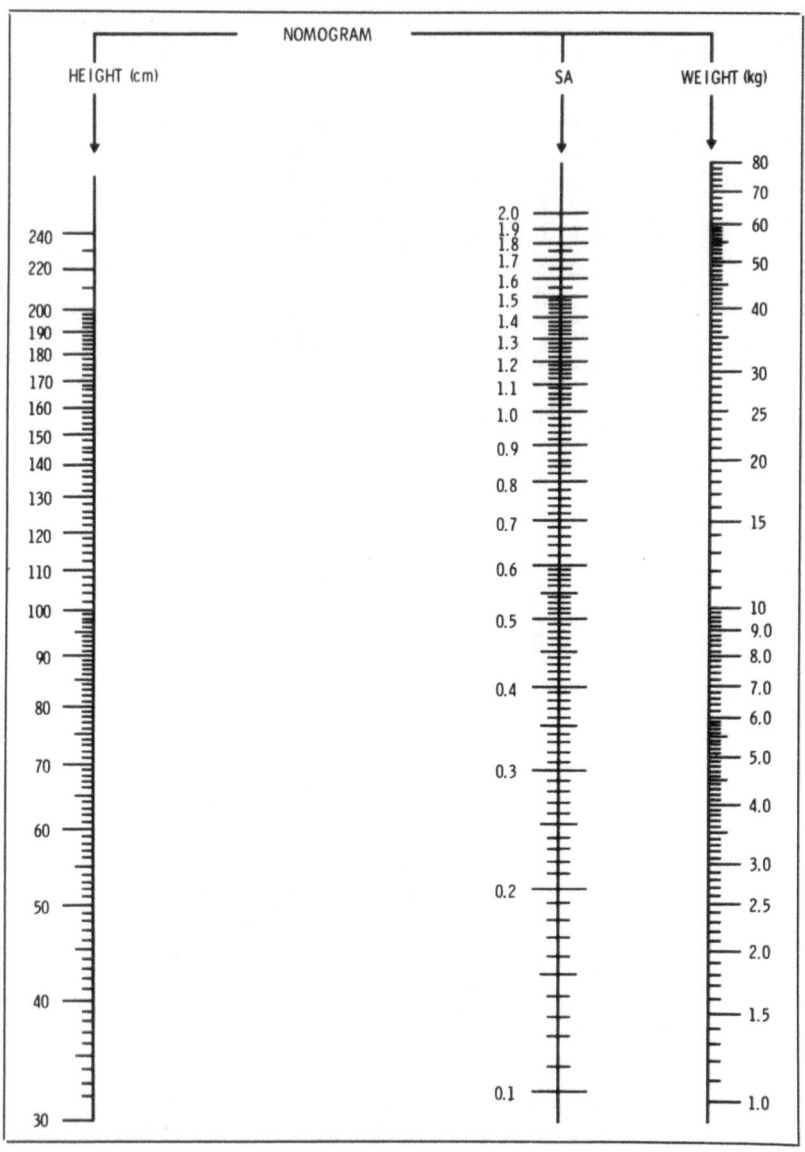

Nomogram to calculate the surface area of a child

Table 2   Doses of antibiotics in neonates (born at term)

Drug	Route	0–7 days old		7–14 days old		Remarks
		Times daily	Dose	Times daily	Dose	
Amikacin	i.m. i.v.	2	7.5 mg/kg	3	7.5 mg/kg	Side-effects and monitor serum levels as for Gentamicin.
Amoxycillin	i.v. i.m.	2 2	25 mg/kg 50 mg/kg	3 4	25 mg/kg 50 mg/kg	For Group B streptococcal sepsis or meningitis.
Ampicillin	i.v. i.m.	2 2	25 mg/kg 50 mg/kg	3 4	25 mg/kg 50 mg/kg	For Group B streptococcal sepsis or meningitis.
Azlocillin	i.v.	2	100 mg/kg	3 4	100 mg/kg if <2.0 kg 100 mg|kg if >2.0 kg	
Carbenicillin	i.v.	2	100 mg/kg	3 4	100 mg/kg if <2.0 kg 100 mg/kg if >2.0 kg	
Cefuroxime	i.v. i.m.	2	20 mg/kg	3	20 mg/kg	
Cephalothin	i.v. i.m.	2	20 mg/kg	3	20 mg/kg	
Chloramphenicol	i.v.	2	12.5 mg/kg	2	12.5–25 mg/kg	Monitor serum levels. May cause the 'grey-baby syndrome'.
Co-trimoxazole (Septrin, Bactrim)	i.v.	2	24 mg/kg	2	24 mg/kg	Avoid if baby is jaundiced.
Flucloxacillin or cloxacillin	i.v.	2	25 mg/kg	3	25 mg/kg	

| Drug | Route | 0–7 days old | | 7–14 days old | | Remarks |
		Times daily	Dose	Times daily	Dose	
Gentamicin	i.m. i.v.	3	2 mg/kg	3	2.5 mg/kg	May be ototoxic or nephrotoxic. Monitor serum levels.
Isoniazid	oral	Single	10 mg/kg	Single	10 mg/kg	
Methicillin	i.v.	2	25 mg/kg if < 2.0 kg	2	25 mg/kg if < 2.0 kg	
		3	25 mg/kg if > 2.0 kg	3	25 mg/kg if > 2.0 kg	
Penicillin G (benzyl penicillin)	i.v. i.m.	2	15 mg/kg	3	15 mg/kg	
		2	30–45 mg/kg	4	25–35 mg/ kg	For group B streptococcal sepsis or meningitis.
Tobramycin	i.m. i.v.	2	2 mg/kg	3	2 mg/kg	Side-effects and monitor serum levels as for Gentamicin

Further details may be found in *Antimicrobial Therapy for Newborns* by McCracken, G., and Nelson, J. D., 1977, Grune and Stratton, New York.

Index

317